THE NEW PRESCRIPTION
MARIJUANA AS MEDICINE

D0792653

Martin Martinez
Edited by Francis Podrebarac, M.D.

Published by Quick American Archives
Oakland, California
www.quicktrading.com

Copyright © 2000 Martin Martinez

The New Prescription: Marijuana As Medicine
ISBN: 0-932551-35-1

Project Manager: S. Rose
Indexing: Shelli Newhart
Copyeditor: Judith Bess
Cover Design & Layout: B. Vallem
Cover Photography: M. Gordon

The New Prescription contains references to published scientific research on the uses of marijuana as medicine. This information is provided for educational purposes, and is not intended as medical advice on any specific condition. This is not a book of approved medical therapies. The author has attempted to illuminate this subject with medical accuracy at the date of publication. As medical research and practices advance, however, therapeutic use and standards may change. It is recommended that patients follow the advice of physicians directly involved in their care.

Marinol® is a registered trademark of Unimed Pharmaceuticals, Inc.

Publisher's Cataloging-in-Publication *(Provided by Quality Books, Inc.)*

Martinez, Martin.
      The new prescription : marijuana as medicine /
      Martin Martinez ; edited by Francis Podrebarac. --
      1st ed.
      p. cm.
      Includes bibliographical references and index.
      ISBN: 0-932551-35-1

      1. Marijuana--Therapeutic use.
      I. Podrebarac, Francis. II. Title.

      RM666.C266 2000   615'.7827
                              QBI00-25

THE NEW PRESCRIPTION
MARIJUANA
AS MEDICINE

Quick American Archives

TABLE OF CONTENTS

Modern Uses of Marijuana as Medicine (Continued)

Modern Uses of Marijuana as Medicine (Continued)

FOREWORD

Physicians in the United States are not trained in the medical uses of marijuana. Instead, we are taught the federal government's political position that marijuana is a Schedule I drug having no medical use whatsoever, and that marijuana is a dangerous, highly addictive "gateway" drug leading to a downward spiral of drug abuse. This book examines evidence that those icons of drug war rhetoric could not be further from the truth.

I learned about the medical uses of marijuana the hard way. In 1995, I was admitted to a hospital severely anemic, dehydrated, and malnourished. A widespread malignant cancer in my intestines and lymph nodes had caused me to lose fifty pounds. The diagnosis was intestinal Kaposi's Sarcoma due to HIV disease. In other words, I had intestinal cancer caused by the deadly AIDS virus. My condition required immediate stabilization because I was literally bleeding and starving to death at the same time. I had no energy, no appetite, severe nausea, vomiting, diarrhea, and constant unimaginable abdominal pain. Intravenous fluids were my only source of sustenance.

My oncologist (cancer specialist) advised me that radiation therapy and surgery were not reasonable treatment options because of the location and extent of cancerous development in my body. She advised that my only hope for survival was chemotherapy; I might live a few more years by regaining my appetite while trying to keep down 25-30 nauseating pills per day. Standard nausea medications, including Compazine and Marinol, were found to be ineffective and caused adverse effects. Desperate for any remedy to my fatal condition, I tried smoking marijuana, which to my surprise benefited my survival in many ways. Marijuana reduced the frequency, duration, and severity of my abdominal pain better than morphine and without the nausea and sedation typical of opiate narcotics. Marijuana reduced my nausea and improved my appetite, enabling me to tolerate chemotherapy and, subsequently, to keep down the so-called "AIDS cocktail" totaling more than 10,000 pills per year. Most importantly, because I smoked the marijuana, the medicinal compounds bypassed my cancerous intestines. Inhalation through my lungs directly into my bloodstream resulted in rapid relief of symptoms with exact control of dosage. I experienced no adverse effects, and no hallucinations or other perceptual disorders, contrary to what I had been led to expect.

Under US law, a Schedule I drug is defined as having a high potential for abuse and no accepted medical use. Schedule I drugs are deemed unsafe for use even under medical supervision. The 1999 Institute of Medicine (IOM) report assessing the scientific base of medical marijuana found that it did not meet any part of that legal definition. The IOM report concluded that accumulated scientific data indicates potential therapeutic value for marijuana in a variety of illnesses, and a lesser potential for drug abuse than commonly prescribed opiates and benzodiazepines—including Valium. Adverse effects of marijuana were found to be within the range tolerated for other medications. The government-sponsored IOM report also debunked the so-called "gateway theory" that marijuana leads to abuse of harder drugs. Rather, the IOM report implicated alcohol and tobacco use by minors as gateways to illicit drug abuse.

More than ten years earlier, in 1988, an elaborate two-year hearing by the Drug Enforcement Administration (DEA) into the medical uses of marijuana came to similar conclusions when DEA Administrative Law Judge Francis Young recommended rescheduling marijuana for medical use. It was Young's determination that there are accepted medical uses for marijuana in the treatment of a variety of diseases, and it was found to be "one of the safest substances known to man." Since then, The New England Journal of Medicine, the world's most prestigious medical research journal, has published multiple editorials calling for the rescheduling of marijuana for medical use. The list of other medical authorities that have endorsed rescheduling marijuana for medical use includes dozens of well-respected national organizations.

For more than 5,000 years marijuana has been used medicinally to treat a variety of ailments without causing a single human death. Ironically, our "new prescription" of marijuana as medicine concerns the oldest known herbal medication. Prior to prohibition of it in 1937, the medical use of marijuana, more properly known as cannabis, was strongly supported by the American Medical Association and prescribed by physicians throughout the country and around the world. While American medical experts petition the government for legal access, cannabis continues to be prescribed in a number of other countries. Recent research points to the natural occurrence of cannabinoid receptors in the human brain and nervous system. Cannabinoids appear to have a natural role in pain modulation, movement, and immune responses to injury. This may explain why there is such overwhelming anecdotal evidence that marijuana brings symptomatic relief to a variety of patients and illnesses.

Sir William Osler (1849-1919) is called the father of modern medicine and the most influential physician in history. He is credited with leading a generation of young doctors away from textbooks and directly to the bedsides of patients. And in spite of this commitment, Osler wrote a medical textbook that was frequently revised and considered authoritative for more than 30 years. He is quoted as saying, "the study of medicine begins with the patient, continues with the patient, and ends with the patient."

Current US policy makers have completely lost sight of this focus on the patient as central to the study of medicine, discounting large numbers of reports from patients—and doctors—as "anecdotal evidence," and therefore unscientific. Yet anecdotal evidence remains as important today as it has been throughout the history of medicine. Anecdotal evidence leads to the restriction of drugs and to their withdrawal from the market; as when Thalidomide was found to cause birth defects, and when the Fen-Phen combination was found to cause heart valve problems. Anecdotal evidence often leads to new uses for a medication; for example, the notorious morning sickness drug, Thalidomide, is now used for treatment of cancer and leprosy, and the anticonvulsant drug, Tegretol, is now used to treat seizures, chronic pain, and bipolar disorder. Anecdotal evidence may prompt a physician to alter a dosage, change medications, or discontinue a medication, based solely on the individual responses of any given patient. With all due respect to the Office of National Drug Control Policy, the wealth of anecdotal evidence supporting marijuana in medical use far outweighs the erroneous legal definition of marijuana as a Schedule I substance.

The author, Martin Martinez, has spent years gathering the facts and compiling the latest research on the medical uses of marijuana, as well as providing an overview of the rich history of this amazing medicine. I hope the reader finds this book as interesting, enlightening, and educational as I have while editing the text for medical accuracy.

FRANCIS PODREBARAC, M.D.

ACKNOWLEDGMENTS

The original version of this book was a Community Service project performed in lieu of a jail sentence to satisfy felony charges of "manufacturing marijuana." This unusual outcome resulted from the author's second arrest for growing medicine, less than two months after his medical necessity trial ended in a hung jury, eight to four in favor of acquittal. Without the cooperation of the Prosecuting Attorney, this book might never have been born. Because that cooperation was heavily influenced by hundreds of marijuana activists in Washington and other states, those fine folks, including the Green Cross Patient Co-operative and the Seattle Hempfest Volunteer Staff, deserve a great share of gratitude. The original version was compiled for the Washington Hemp Education Network, headed by Bob Owen and Dave Edwards, M.D., who provided the legal means to avoid imprisonment.

While clearly imperfect and regionally interpreted, state laws protecting medical marijuana patients may serve to prevent such painful demonstrations of suffering in the future. All those who have helped signal a new understanding of marijuana, if only by their vote, are also to be thanked for moral support. Individuals and organizations who have provided the essential material of this book are listed in the Bibliography and Notes sections. Obviously, this book would not exist were it not for those thousands of people who have worked to promote honest and intelligent information on medical marijuana.

ACKNOWLEDGEMENTS

Francis Podrebarac, M.D. provided an educated ear and technical criticism essential to the factual articulation of many passages. Lester Grinspoon, M.D. offered encouragement and inspiration. Members of Hemp-talk@hemp.net supplied additional research. John Stahl helped prepare the original manuscript. John Stuart told me what he liked about the book. Judith Bess told me what was wrong with it. Andy McBeth, Stephanie Rose and the staff of Quick American Archives were most supportive and shaped the presentation to its present state.

Along with many unnamed supporters, this work was made possible with the assistance of my co-defendant, Danielle Brooke.

INTRODUCTION

A Brief History of Medical Marijuana

M any civilizations throughout history have had a powerful dependence on hemp, mankind's most durable natural fiber resource. While modern-day proponents of industrial hemp often distance these uses of the plant from the drug called marijuana, the two terms—*hemp* and *marijuana*—apply to different uses of the same plant species. A history of marijuana as medicine would be incomplete without some reference to the multitude of benefits provided by this extraordinary weed.

The earliest known evidence of marijuana in human hands dates back approximately 10,000 years to a prehistoric village that was discovered in Taiwan in 1972. Pottery shards unearthed there bore the distinct impression of hemp cord, conclusively proving that marijuana has been in use since the Stone Age.

Known in Chinese languages as *Ma*, this hardy annual herb is arguably the "mother" of agricultural civilization. *Ma* provided to be a renewable food source and a durable textile fiber for the manufacture of rope and fabric, setting agro-industrial China far ahead of hunter-gatherer tribes in other parts of the world. Besides its many textile and medicinal uses, marijuana yields seeds rich in B vitamins, protein, and amino acids, which have served as China's second or third most important agricultural food source for thousands of years.

While evidence of marijuana in use as a medicine has been found in Egyptian ruins dated as early as the 16th century BC, and digs at ancient Hebrew sites have unearthed evidence of medical marijuana as an aid to childbirth long before the time of Christ, the many uses of *Ma* have proved to be an invaluable resource in the continuous survival of Chinese culture from its distant origins to the present day.

The earliest known material identified as hemp fabric was found in an ancient burial site from the Chou Dynasty (1122-1249 BC), confirming numerous historical references to the importance of hemp in early China. In the *Book of Rites* (circa 200 BC) mourners were instructed to wear hemp fabric out of respect for the dead, a tradition which survives to this day.

Perhaps most importantly, the Chinese invention of hemp paper around 200 BC revolutionized record-keeping processes fundamental to orderly government. Although the secret was kept from the rest of the world for 900 years, hemp papermaking eventually became indispensable to the rapid development of all civilizations throughout the world. Thousands of years before hemp paper became a central fixture of European civilizations, the industrial and medical uses of *Ma* were deeply rooted in China, the country historically known as "the land of mulberry and hemp."

In ancient China, medicine men used hemp stalks carved with ornate snake figures as magical amulets to exorcise demons believed to be the cause of physical illnesses. These healers attempted to cure all sorts of diseases by beating the headboards of their patients' beds with magical hemp stalks while reciting spells and incantations. Japanese Shinto Priests employed a similar ceremony using a short wand bound with undyed hemp fibers. The purity of white hemp was thought to exorcise evil demons. While contemporary scientists dismiss such accounts as ignorant superstitions, a more thoughtful observer might ponder the origins of such long-lived legends.

Shen-Nung, a Chinese emperor who ruled around 2800 BC, is credited with introducing medicines to the Chinese people. Like all mythic figures, he is recalled through time in both fact and fantasy. It is said that Shen-Nung had a transparent abdomen and intentionally ingested as many as 70 different plants per day so that he could watch their effects and discover their various qualities. Shen-Nung identified hundreds of different medicines, which are compiled in the world's oldest medical text, the *Pen Ts'ao*. For that he was deified and is still acclaimed as the father of traditional Chinese medicine. Prior to the reorganization of China as a communist country, medicinal drug retailers offered periodic discounts in honor of Shen-Nung.

According to the *Pen Ts'ao, ma-fen*, the flowers of the female marijuana plant, contain the greatest amount of *yin* energy: *yin* being the receptive female attribute that is, in traditional Chinese philosophy and medicine, dynamically linked with *yang*, the creative male element. *Ma-fen* was prescribed in cases of a loss of *yin*, such as in menstrual fatigue, rheumatism, malaria, beri-beri, constipation, and absentmindedness. The *Pen Ts'ao* warned that eating too many *Ma* seeds could cause one to see demons, but that, taken over a long period of time, marijuana seeds could enable one to communicate with spirits. Shen-Nung also instructed the Chinese people in the cultivation of hemp for clothing and other textile uses, an agricultural art still practiced in rural areas of China.

In the first century AD, Taoist alchemists inhaled the smoke of burning hemp seeds in order to cause visions, which were valued as a means of achieving immortality. Marijuana was considered a superior elixir that rejuvenated the mind and body. In more pragmatic disciplines, traditional Chinese physicians have used *ma* for a wide variety of medical conditions. Hua T'o, a famous surgeon of the second century AD, performed complicated surgery using *ma-yo*, an anesthetic made from hemp resin and wine. When acupuncture and medicines failed to effect a cure, Hua T'o performed complex surgery, including amputations and organ graftings tied with sutures. With the use of *ma-yo*, these surgeries were reportedly painless. In the tenth century AD, Chinese physicians reported that *ma-yo* was useful in the treatment of waste diseases and injuries. *Ma* treatments were used to clear the blood and cool fevers, as well as to cure rheumatism and to ease childbirth.

In Western civilizations, as in China, the durable material crafted from tough hemp stalks has been of immeasurable significance throughout history. The ancient Greeks called it *kannabis*. Greek sailors traded *kannabis* across the Aegean Sea as early as the sixth century BC, according to written records on hemp trade from that era. Twentieth-century archeologists found hemp fiber bundles in the cargo hold of a Carthaginian trade ship that had sunk near Sicily around 300 BC. In 450 BC, Herodotus, the great Greek historian, wrote of the fine quality of hemp clothing produced by the Greek-speaking Thracians.

Four hundred years later, Plutarch wrote that the Thracians made a habit of throwing the tops of the *kannabis* plant onto a fire, thereby becoming intoxicated by the smoke. It was a custom unfamiliar to the wine-loving children of Zeus. A minor reference to the use of *kannabis* as a remedy for backache is found in Greek literature from about 400 BC. That is the only known reference to the medical use of marijuana in ancient Greece, although it is known that both Arabic and Hebrew medical practices did use *kannabis* medications during that same period.

In 70 AD, a Greek physician named Discordes in the employ of conquering Roman legions collected a wealth of information on medicinal plants. Discordes' text, entitled *Materia Medica*, contained the fruits of his world travels with the Roman armies. He listed 600 medicinal plants, complete with descriptions, local names, natural habitats, and indications for treatment of various symptoms. Among those 600 plants Discordes identified *Cannabis sativa L.* (from the Greek *kannabis*) as being useful in manufacturing rope and as producing seeds whose juice was effective for treating earaches and for diminishing sexual desire. Discordes' *Materia Medica* was hugely successful, translated into every language of the known world, and remained an indispensable reference manual of Western medicine for at least 1500 years.

The English word *canvas* is derived from the word *cannabis*, an etymological indication of the supreme importance of hemp fiber in European seafaring technology. Clearly, the colonial expansion of European empires into remote parts of the world could not have occurred without the development of cannabis-based technologies. In 1492, for example, each one of Columbus' transatlantic vessels carried more than 80 tons of hemp rigging and sails, the product of untold thousands of man-hours. Many stately fortunes were built on the toil of peasants in tall fields of hemp, which eventually became the most important industrial crop in most emerging countries. At the same time, European knowledge of medical cannabis was limited to the short references of Discordes and various unrecorded folk remedies throughout medieval times.

As Western civilization moved from the Dark Ages into the Renaissance period, the developing medical science uncovered many substantial facts, including a remarkable number of benefits ascribed to medical marijuana. In 1621, in *The Anatomy of Melancholy*, Robert Burton suggested that cannabis might be useful for treating depression. In 1682, *The New London Dispensatory* briefly covered the use of cannabis seeds to cure coughs and jaundice. *The New English Dispensatory* of 1764 recommended boiling hemp roots and applying the poultice to reduce inflammation. *The Edinburg New Dispensary* of 1794 reported an increased understanding of the medicinal uses of the cannabis plant, including the treatment of coughs, venereal disease, and urinary incontinence. The section on cannabis notes that "Although the seeds only have hitherto been principally in use, yet other parts of the plant seem to be more active, and may be considered as deserving more attention." In 1814, Nicholas Culpepper published his *Complete Herbal*, which listed all of the known medicinal uses of cannabis. He included all of the applications previously published and a few new ones, such as easing colic, allaying humors of the bowels, staying troublesome bleeding, reducing inflammation of the head, and reducing pains of the hips and joints. Culpepper also recommended cannabis as an additive to salves in the treatment of burns. There is no historical evidence that European physicians were aware of any psychoactive effects associated with cannabis use until the exploration of India broadened European understanding.

In 1753 a Swedish botanist named Carl Lineaus compiled the most complete reference manual of botanical classifications to date, entitled *Species Planetarium*. Linaeus adopted Discordes' classification of *Cannabis sativa*, but almost immediately some botanists argued that the newly studied Indian cannabis plant was distinctly different from the well-known European Cannabis sativa grown for industrial and medical uses. In 1783, a French biologist named Jean Lamarck examined the two types in his compendium entitled *Encyclopedia*. Lamarck noted that the species *Cannabis sativa* commonly grown for fiber and textile uses was characterized by a height of twelve to sixteen feet, long stalks, sparse foliage, and slender leaves. Cannabis native to India, on the other hand, was typically four to five feet tall at maturity and was densely foliated with bushy clusters of comparatively broad leaves. Lamarck dubbed the second species *Cannabis indica* in deference to its country of origin.

There are literally hundreds of subspecies of cannabis, and botanists continue to argue over exact scientific classifications, but most experts concur that there are at least two distinctly different types comprising all of the strains currently in existence. In 1913, Lyster Dewey, botanist and hemp expert from the United States Department of Agriculture, reported in the *USDA Yearbook* that *Cannabis indica* was " . . . different in general appearance from any of the numerous forms grown by this department from seed obtained in nearly all countries where hemp is cultivated."

Modern hybridization has altered the natural inclinations of the cannabis plant as growers have sought to promote particular traits, blurring distinction between the two primary species. However, those natural tendencies remain at least partially visible. Typically, the tall stalks of *Cannabis sativa* are cultivated for fiber and seed industries, while the short *Cannabis indica* bushes are cultivated for the medicinal and psychoactive properties of their flowers. *Cannabis sativa* grown for industrial uses usually contains only minor amounts of psychoactive compounds. Proper cultivation can produce higher levels of therapeutic compounds in some types of *Cannabis sativa*. The more potent *Cannabis indica* varieties, on the other hand, are not suitable for industrial fiber production due to the shortness of their bushy stalks. While this contrast distinguishes the natural tendencies of the two primary varieties, many medicinal growers have discovered that the most potent strains combine the best traits of both.

Apparently originating in China, cannabis presumably spread west across Asia, Asia Minor, and the Mediterranean, and was adopted by many early cultures. From there, cannabis eventually spread to nearly all civilizations around the globe, according to Western historians. Traditional Hindu teachings, however, tell an entirely different story. The origins of what Europeans called *Cannabis indica* are recorded in the *Vedas*, India's four most sacred books. Written approximately 4,000 years ago, the Vedas tell the great legends of conquest, struggle, and spiritual development that continue to shape every facet of traditional Hindu life. Among many other colorful myths, the Vedas tell of Lord Shiva, one of three primary Hindu gods, refreshed in the heat of the day by eating leaves of the marijuana plant. Lord Shiva adopted it as his favorite food; hence he is honored with the title Lord of *Bhang*.

Bhang is a traditional Indian beverage made of cannabis mixed with various herbs and spices, which has been popular in India for ages. *Bhang* is a less powerful preparation than *Ganja*, which is prepared from flowering plants for smoking and eating. *Charas*, more potent than either *Bhang* or *Ganja*, consists of cannabis flower tops harvested at full bloom. Dense with sticky resin, *Charas* is nearly as potent as the concentrated cannabis resin preparations called *hashish*. For thousands of years these intoxicating marijuana preparations have permeated every important aspect of traditional Indian life, from ritualistic worship to mundane survival. Warriors preparing for battle, couples about to wed, and pious Hindus on virtually every important occasion have celebrated life by invoking Lord Shiva with the sacred herb.

The fourth book of the *Vedas*, the *Athavaveda*, which is translated as *The Science of Charms*, calls Bhang one of the "five kingdoms of herbs . . . which releases us from anxiety." While this idea may appear to echo Western understandings, South Asian wisdom is not bound by the limits of Newtonian logic. One Hindu myth tells of the time before creation when the gods churned the great cosmic mountain for the nectar of immortality. It is said that marijuana plants sprouted wherever the precious drops of nectar touched the earth. Another mystical *sutra* reports that Siddhartha, he who became known as Buddha, "the enlightened one," lived on nothing but a single cannabis seed per day for six years prior to his spiritual awakening. While a literal interpretation is not possible, these ancient myths do remind us that both Hindus and Tantric Buddhists in Northern India, Tibet, and Nepal have included cannabis as an essential sacrament in profound religious rituals for untold millennia.

Traditional Indian medicine has long used a multitude of cannabis preparations for the treatment of such illnesses as fever, dysentery, sunstroke, and leprosy. Cannabis is said to clear phlegm, quicken digestion, sharpen the intellect, increase the body's alertness, and act as an *elixir vitae*. Hindu medical practice—unlike Western science—also addresses spiritual awareness. It is said that *Ganja* gives delight to Shiva, the king of gods, who is always pleased to receive offerings. This connection between Lord Shiva and *Ganja* is considered invaluable to maintaining one's physical health and psychological equilibrium. According to the *Rajvallabha*, a 17th century Hindu text, "This desire-fulfilling drug was believed to have been obtained by men on Earth for the welfare of all people. To those who use it regularly, it begets joy and diminishes sorrow."

Indian culture reveres the marijuana plant as a sacrament and a blessing. Through it one may partake of cosmic forces and unite with the gods. Although Western societies typically reject subjective spiritual experiences, the importance of these beliefs in Indian culture cannot be discounted. In 1893, after exhaustive study of cannabis use in their South Asian colony, the British government released the largest single study of cannabis use to date in the *Indian Hemp Drugs Commission Report*. Years of research produced the official determination that the use of hemp drugs was not harmful to the Indians, and that it would be a grievous error to attempt to separate that culture from the holy drug known to the West as *Cannabis indica*. In 1986, however, the Single Convention on Drugs and Narcotic Substances outlawed cannabis throughout the world. The current ban includes African, Asian, Middle Eastern, and South American countries whose history of cannabis use was also of great social and cultural significance long before the arrival of hemp-heavy warships from faraway lands.

During the early days of the American colonies, industrial hemp products became indispensable to world trade. Hemp was a government-mandated crop, yet the many medical uses of the marijuana plant remained largely unknown in both the Old and the New World. However, once Westerners discovered the range of cannabis therapies found in traditional Indian medicine, the effects of *Cannabis indica* on European and American medical practices were swift and strong.

In the 19th century, after extensive study of the Indian medical literature, and after discussing cannabis with many Indian scholars, the British East India Company surgeon William B. O'Shoughnessy began testing *Cannabis indica* on animals and patients, and also on himself. O'Shoughnessy introduced many new medicinal uses of cannabis to Europe and America in his 1839 paper titled *On the Preparation of the*

Indian Hemp or Gunja. O'Shoughnessy found that cannabis relieved rheumatism, convulsions, and muscle spasms of tetanus and rabies. That original medical research remains a historical record calling for further scrutiny in our current postindustrial era.

Following O'Shoughnessy's work, the late 1800s saw a rapid increase of cannabis therapies in Western medical practice. In 1840, French physician Louis Aubert-Roche published a book on the use of hashish to treat symptoms of the plague and typhoid fever. In 1854 the United States Dispensatory listed many uses of cannabis extracts, recommending cannabis preparations for cases of neuralgia, gout, tetanus, hydrophobia, cholera, convulsions, spasticity, hysteria, depression, insanity, and uterine hemorrhage, and also for promoting relaxed contractions during delivery.

In 1890 Sir John Russell Reynolds, personal physician to Queen Victoria, reported that cannabis was useful for treatment of dysmenorrhea (painful menstruation), migraine, neuralgia, convulsions, and insomnia. Reynolds called cannabis "by far the most useful of drugs" in treating "painful maladies." It is unknown whether Reynolds or other Western physicians knew of the corroborating recommendations written by China's Shen Nung more than two thousand years earlier.

Between 1840 and 1890 at least 100 medical papers were published on the uses of cannabis for the treatment of loss of appetite, insomnia, migraine headache, pain, involuntary twitching, excessive coughing, and withdrawal in cases of opiate or alcohol addiction. Sir William Osler, known as "the father of modern medicine," proclaimed cannabis to be the best treatment for migraine in his authoritative medical textbook written in 1915. At that time, there were at least 30 different cannabis preparations made by leading pharmaceutical companies available in America, even though the hypodermic injection of morphine, along with the use of aspirin and other medicines, had already begun to replace traditional herbal medications.

INTRODUCTION

George Washington, Thomas Jefferson, and other founding fathers had repeatedly extolled the many virtues of hemp, but their words were quickly discounted as the industrial revolution radically reinvented American values. Domestic policies driven by capitalistic motives and a marked prejudice against people of color, the primary users of cannabis as a "recreational" drug, led to the 1937 Marijuana Tax Act, a bill that effectively outlawed all uses of hemp by the imposition of a cost-prohibitive tax.

During the closed congressional hearings of 1937 the American Medical Association adamantly objected to the prohibition of medical marijuana. The testimony of the Association's legislative counsel, Dr. William C. Woodward, in response to the one-sided testimony of career-minded law enforcers, heatedly criticized the proceedings and their determined intent. He told the legislators:

> In all that you have heard here thus far, no mention has been made of any excessive use of the drug by any doctor or its excessive distribution by any pharmacist. And yet the burden of this bill is placed heavily upon the doctors and pharmacists of the country, and I may say very heavily-most heavily possibly of all-on farmers of the country.
>
> We cannot understand yet, Mr. Chairman, why this bill should have been prepared in secret for two years, without any initiative, even to the profession that it was being prepared. No medical man would identify this bill with a medicine until he read it through, because *marijuana* is not a drug ... simply a name given to cannabis.

Misrepresenting a standard medication that had been used in medical practice for nearly a century by incorporating a Mexican slang word, *marihuana*, the 1937 Tax Act was a classic example of what social critic Noam Chomsky calls "manufacturing consent." The committee was unabashed in its mockery of the democratic process. For his directness and honesty, Dr. Woodward was rewarded with the following admonition:

> You are not cooperative in this. If you want to advise us on legislation you ought to come here with some constructive proposals rather than criticisms, rather than trying to throw obstacles in the way of something the Federal government is trying to do.

Regardless of the interests of the American Medical Association and numerous pharmaceutical companies such as Parke-Davis and Ely Lilly, and with no consideration of various hemp fiber industries, including the Ford Corporation and thousands of American farmers, the United States government effectively banned cannabis use for all purposes. The move was apparently based solely on the lies of certain federal law enforcers who were backed by newspaper magnate William Randolph Hearst. Hearst stirred hysteria in the country about an evil drug known as "the weed with roots in hell." Having little or no experience with the mysterious *marihuana* plant, most Americans were easily duped by Hearst's blatant fabrications. Few were even aware of the great loss to medical science. In retrospect, it is clear that the outrageous stories of murder and mayhem widely publicized throughout the country were intended to destroy the hemp industry because it posed a threat to tree-paper industrialist Hearst and synthetic-fiber industrialist Dupont, among others. Just as the vast fortunes of European courts were built on the backs of hemp farmers, so were modern industrial fortunes built on their destruction. Not to be outdone by the private sector, politicians and law enforcers secured a whole new frontier for themselves by banning one of humanity's most precious medicinal herbs.

Cannabis remained legally prescribable until 1942, but its medical use had dwindled by that time because of the exorbitant tax on *marihuana*. During those years, *Reefer Madness* propaganda helped erase America's cultural memory of hemp, the material on which both the Declaration of Independence and the US Constitution were originally written. During World War II, the industrial uses of hemp fiber were hugely promoted by the US government to outfit American armies overseas, but at the close of the war, the patriotic "Hemp for Victory" slogan became yet another bit of hemp trivia quietly deleted from America's official history. Although America's industrial hero, Henry Ford, had created a car made of hemp that was harder than steel, his great ingenuity was quickly forgotten, as was our age-old reliance on one of nature's greatest medicines.

Scientific study of cannabis and its many medical applications was minimal for several decades. While there were over 2500 papers on opiate drugs published between 1938 and 1965, there were only 175 studies of cannabis during the same period. Enforced ignorance prevailed until the cultural revolution of the 1960s focused a new light on the subject.

The Renaissance of Cannabis Consciousness

The popularity of marijuana among dissenting American youths during the 1960s triggered a resurgence of scientific research, but federal mandates soon made unbiased study nearly impossible. While President Kennedy purportedly used cannabis in the White House to relieve severe back pain, subsequent Presidents radically escalated US "drug war" policies. Richard Nixon promised to get tough on drugs during his presidential campaign, and he kept that promise almost immediately upon assuming office. He appointed the Shafer Commission to study the "marijuana problem," but the President's commission determined that major problems associated with marijuana use were largely the result of its prohibition. Discovering that the report backed decriminalization, Nixon rejected his commission's recommendations before they were published. When framed by law enforcers, high-profile Harvard professor and professional dropout Timothy Leary successfully challenged the faulty logic of the

1937 Marijuana Tax Act. Nixon quickly rewrote the nation's drug laws, and Leary went to prison. The Controlled Substances Act of 1970 classified marijuana as a Schedule I drug with "no medical value and a high potential for abuse," and thus created severe obstacles to objective research.

For three decades, countless politicians relied on drug war rhetoric to maintain their positions. President Jimmy Carter was the only prominent US policy maker to even consider revising the nation's marijuana laws, and even that consideration was short lived. Enforcing cannabis prohibition has cost inestimable billions of US tax dollars. Millions of American citizens have suffered physical, mental, economic, and social hardship resulting from the political ambitions of politicians and law enforcement officials. In 1997, the editor-in-chief of the widely respected *New England Journal of Medicine* coined the term "federal foolishness" in criticizing the government's persecution of 65 million Americans.

Among the millions of confessed criminals, both President Bill Clinton and his one-time nemesis Speaker of the House Newt Gingrich have admitted to using cannabis for recreational purposes. Nonetheless, both the Republican and Democratic parties prospered defending the country against its fourth most popular drug, jailing over half a million people per year. For American doctors and their patients, conversations regarding marijuana were strictly limited by the legal definition of marijuana as a substance of abuse. But, regardless of harsh penalties, social stigma, and enforced ignorance, popular interest in the "forbidden medicine" has dramatically increased. At the dawn of the new millennium, ancient wisdom has become modern folklore.

In the age of AIDS and Cancer chemotherapy, cannabis has assumed a powerful stature in public opinion. In July of 1998, a stunning 96% of respondents supported the medical use of marijuana, according to a CNN news poll headlined "Weed Wars: A Smoldering Debate Enters the Mainstream." Also in 1998, the Microsoft News Broadcasting Service poll showed 90% public acceptance of medical marijuana. While CBS reported only 65% approval in 1997, 20% of those polled thought that medical marijuana should be legalized even if research failed to confirm anecdotal reports. The American Civil Liberties Union poll of 1996 found that 79% of Americans thought it would be a "good idea" to allow doctors to prescribe cannabis, and 25% of those polled reported knowing a friend or relative who had used marijuana for medical purposes. Those national polls all preceded the Institute of Medicine (IOM) report, *Marijuana and Medicine: Assessing the Science Base,* in 1999 (see appendix). Following release of that landmark federal review, a Gallop poll found that 73% of the American people support "making marijuana available for doctors to prescribe in order to reduce pain and suffering."

Tens of thousands of seriously ill Americans are now physician-certified users of medical marijuana. Many states have legalized the use of marijuana when recommended by a physician, and at least 20 other states have contemplated similar referenda. But the popular movement to legalize medical marijuana is severely crippled by hypocritical "federal foolishness." Although a mountain of overwhelming evidence supports the safety and utility of medical marijuana, it remains a Schedule I substance, along with LSD, PCP, methamphetamines, heroin, and other dangerous drugs. Regardless of the will of the people, as expressed in numerous statewide ballot initiatives, federal law is enforced throughout the nation.

Marinol, an oral pharmaceutical medication containing the most prominent cannabinoid, delta-9 tetrahydrocannibinol, (THC) is legally available by prescription for appetite stimulation in treating anorexic AIDS patients, and for the control of nausea in cancer chemotherapy. And the use of Marinol in cancer treatment and in the growing AIDS crisis has helped pave the way for recognition of marijuana in other fields of medical practice.

But challenges to intelligent discussion remain daunting. Cannabis cooperatives distribute the natural medication to qualified patients in many North American cities, defiant of federal court orders. Even in states that have enacted laws protecting qualified patients from prosecution, law enforcement authorities, traditional enemies of "demon weed," have no protocol covering the growing presence of medical cannabis—a hydra of multiplying complications. At stake in this multifaceted contest are the rights of life, liberty, and the pursuit of happiness: in particular, patients' rights, physicians' rights of free speech, the rights of the disabled, and the sovereign rights of individual states that have approved the use of medical marijuana in violation of federal law. Landmark legal cases are headlined while top-level drug warriors terrorize the public with irrational and inhumane policies. Caught in the crossfire are an increasing number of seriously ill patients who commit felonies on a daily basis as a matter of personal survival.

It is now common knowledge that marijuana has a variety of medical applications. Even the White House Office of National Drug Control Policy has admitted that the evidence for marijuana as medicine is incontrovertible, after decades of staunch denial. Scientific research on cannabis remains incomplete, yet a great body of information may be gathered from diverse sources. In 1993, Peter Nelson of Australia's Advisory Committee on Illicit Drugs conducted a review of the scientific literature. He discovered that at least 4,000 papers, monographs, and books had been published on the medical, psychological, and social aspects of cannabis use since the 1960s. American health authority Andrew Weil has suggested that the available data on cannabis might fill several tractor-trailer containers. In fact, according to Harvard psychiatrist Lester Grinspoon, we now know more about cannabis than about the majority of prescription drugs in common use.

The Compassionate Investigational New Drug program began distributing government-grown marijuana to a handful of medical marijuana patients in 1978. As of this writing, the program still supplies 300 marijuana cigarettes per month to eight surviving patients. In 1992 the program stopped accepting new applications, just as it was about to be inundated by thousands of applicants with AIDS.

Four years later, medical marijuana was legalized in California and Arizona. Because of the medical marijuana initiatives approved in these two states, President Clinton allocated one million dollars to review the existing research. As a result, in 1999, the most respected medical body in the United States, the Institute of Medicine, published *Marijuana and Medicine: Assessing the Science Base*, in which the authors reported that "The accumulated scientific data indicate a potential therapeutic value for cannabinoid drugs, particularly for pain relief, control of nausea and vomiting, and appetite stimulation." The American government had finally granted official recognition of this natural medicinal resource. However, to understate the obvious, there are a number of potential benefits not listed in the Institute of Medicine's report.

Isolation of some of the 61 active compounds found in cannabis resin, known as cannabinoids, has enabled many studies to be done without the use of the natural material, which still remains almost impossible to obtain for legitimate studies. Immediately following the IOM's 1999 report, the White House promised to support independent research on medical marijuana, yet only one such study has been allowed. Volunteer subjects supplying their own marijuana have provided an additional resource for modern research, and studies done in countries more tolerant of cannabis use offer another source of reliable information. Largely suppressed in the United States, an increasing number of scientific reports provide strong evidence of an amazing number of potential medical uses.

The remainder of this book is essentially an alphabetical annotated list of the therapeutic applications of cannabis and cannabinoid compounds indicated by verified anecdotal reports and validated scientific studies collected from reliable sources, primarily in English speaking countries during contemporary times. Included in the list also are some common issues and myths surrounding the use of marijuana. It is the purpose of this book to give the reader easy access to the scientific basis for the use of marijuana as medicine.

MODERN USES
OF MARIJUANA AS
MEDICINE

Acquired Immune Deficiency Syndrome

Acquired Immune Deficiency Syndrome, (AIDS) is caused by the Human Immunodeficiency Virus (HIV). The virus is usually contracted through sexual contact, intravenous needle sharing, maternal transmission to newborns, or transfusion of contaminated blood products. AIDS is now considered the worst plague in human history. The United Nations estimates that more than 30 million people have already contracted the AIDS virus, and 16,000 new victims are infected every day.[1] In the United States, the Centers for Disease Control and Prevention estimates that 235,470 US citizens were living with AIDS in 1996.[2] More than 350,000 Americans have died of the disease since the epidemic began in 1981.[3] Even more alarming, about one-third of infected Americans are unaware that they are carrying the deadly virus.[4]

In January of 1998, *Newsday* reported that Americans over the age of 50 were the highest AIDS risk group of the 1990s. The number of older Americans with AIDS rose at twice the rate of that of younger people from 1991 to 1996. The mortality rate of those cases was twice that of 13- to 49-year-olds.[5] In July of 1998, *ABC News* reported an even greater AIDS risk

21

among African Americans. While African Americans comprise only 13% of the American population, they account for 57% of all new AIDS cases. AIDS is considered the leading cause of death among African Americans aged 25 to 44.[6]

Although the worldwide death toll from AIDS continues to rise sharply, the AIDS mortality rate in the United States actually dropped by 23% in 1996 compared to 1995.[7] There are few studies examining the causes of this decrease.[8] National media sources have been quick to credit new multidrug "cocktails" containing protease inhibitors. Yet a study from the University of California indicates that these drugs are effective for only about half of the patients who use them. UCSF researchers tracking 136 HIV patients at San Francisco General Hospital's AIDS clinic showed a 50% failure rate of protease inhibitor therapy.[9] ACT UP, the national independent AIDS coalition, cites reports in the gay press linking protease inhibitors to anemia, kidney and liver failure, impaired nutrient absorption, and grotesque physical deformities.[10] While some factions of ACT UP espouse extremist theories, the coalition's mistrust of new AIDS medications that have been rushed through the federal approval process is far from groundless. Mounting cases of bizarre disfigurement and increased risk of heart disease among AIDS patients have prompted the US Food and Drug Administration (FDA) to undertake further studies of protease inhibitors, the "lifesaving drugs" that have been widely prescribed since 1996.[11] Most experts believe that protease inhibitors have radically reduced the mortality rate of AIDS patients in the United States. Although the serious side effects may cause some alarm, medical authorities strongly advise AIDS patients receiving protease inhibitor chemotherapy to continue the treatment as advised by their physician. Discontinuing protease therapy leads to the development of highly resistant HIV strains, which become more difficult to treat.[12]

The mounting AIDS crisis, with San Francisco at the epicenter, was the most prominent driving force behind

California's Proposition 215, "The Compassionate Use Act of 1996." The controversial ballot initiative provided an affirmative legal defense to charges of possession and cultivation of marijuana when recommended by a physician. In some northern California counties, the Compassionate Use Act garnered over 70% of the vote. In San Francisco, for example, more votes were cast for legalization of medical marijuana than were cast for reelection of President Clinton. Two months after the law was approved, the US Drug Czar, General Barry McCaffrey, threatened to prosecute doctors who discussed cannabis therapeutics with their patients. California's physicians were then forced to defend their right to recommend medical marijuana, and that right was upheld in Federal Court.[13] Apparently, regardless of federal bully tactics, a large number of doctors believe that cannabis deserves some share of the credit for the decrease of AIDS-related deaths in the United States.

Thousands of people with AIDS have sworn by medical marijuana, both in press reports and in numerous government hearings. Malignant lymphoma is a common ailment in AIDS cases, as is Kaposi's Sarcoma, a rare form of vascular cancer. Both of these cancers have been treated successfully with the adjunctive application of natural cannabis.[14,15] Such cancerous complications are very common in people with AIDS.

More commonly, however, HIV and AIDS patients suffer from severe anorexia. They become unable to eat and frequently drop weight at an alarming pace. This pattern, called "the wasting syndrome," is the major contributor to death through AIDS-related conditions. Cannabis has been known to stimulate the appetite and promote gastrointestinal reflexes since the beginning of recorded civilization. Shen-Nung, the Father of Chinese Medicine, prescribed *Ma* for constipation almost five thousand years ago. In 1814 Nicholas Culpepper wrote that cannabis was useful for "allaying humors of the bowels." Traditional Hindu medicine also credits cannabis with promoting efficient digestion. Western physicians published many studies in the mid- and late 1800s verifying cannabis' remarkable appetite stimulating properties. This universal effect of marijuana became known as "the munchies" in popular vernacular of the 1960s. In modern America, Marinol, a pill containing synthetic THC, the most powerful of 61 naturally occurring cannabinoid compounds, is routinely prescribed for AIDS patients when other medications fail, yet the source of THC, the marijuana plant, is officially classified by the US government as having "no medical value."

Marinol is effective for some but not all AIDS patients. One problem with synthetic THC is its high potency. Marinol is considered about five times more psychoactive than cannabis,[16] often causing intoxication to the point of incapacity or sedation: perplexing to patients attempting to maintain their lifestyles. Because the body's ability to assimilate THC fluctuates throughout the day, a marijuana smoker is better able to accurately judge dose effectiveness and thereby avoid excessive and prolonged intoxication.[17] However, the difference in potency between Marinol and marijuana is not simply a matter of different dosages. Orally ingested THC is assimilated by the liver, producing cannabinoid metabolite by-products that are active intoxicants remaining in the bloodstream for up to 30 hours following ingestion. When marijuana is smoked rather than eaten, the medicinal compounds enter the bloodstream through the respiratory system, bypassing the liver. Smoked marijuana is also less overwhelming than the THC pill because of its natural complexity. Along with tetrahydrocannabinol, marijuana contains other medicinal cannabinoids that are known to offset the overstimulation of pure THC. These complementary cannabinoids are not found in Marinol. The National Academy of Science's Institute of Medicine is one of many medical bodies that have recommended further research on these other cannabinoids,[18] but the huge cost of such research is a major obstacle. Pharmeceutical companies prefer to patent synthetic cannabinoid analogues rather than naturally-occurring cannabinoid compounds that can be produced at home in a small garden.

Many HIV and AIDS patients report that natural cannabis is far more effective than Marinol, and that cannabis relieves not only the deadly "wasting syndrome," but also the side-effects of protease inhibitor therapy, a daily regimen of 25 to 30 powerful chemotherapy drugs that cause severe nausea. One AIDS physician has remarked, "Not only is marijuana the safest drug an AIDS patient takes, inhalation is the perfect delivery system because it is rapidly effective, easy to dose for the individual patient, and it bypasses complicating factors in the digestive tract."[19]

In addition, the Merck guide to pharmaceutical medicines indicates that Marinol has been shown to increase appetite, but research does not indicate that using the Marinol pill actually increases a patient's body mass. Marijuana's effect on increasing body mass is now a subject of comparative study at San Francisco General Hospital.[20]

While the United Nations World Health Organization reports that a 1989 study indicated that continued cannabis use by HIV-positive males did not increase the progression of AIDS,[21] important American studies confirming the medical utility of marijuana have been mired in federal bureaucracy for many years. A study by Donald Abrams, Director of HIV research at San Francisco General Hospital, was designed to compare the medical effectiveness of cannabis with that of Marinol. The first version of that study was submitted for federal approval in 1992. After seven years of rejection, Abrams' research was finally approved only after being modified to test for marijuana's safety rather than its medical effectiveness—a distinction ensuring that the study would be ineligible as a test of medical effectiveness required for FDA approval.[22] After two more years of federal hurdles, the National Institutes of Health allowed Dr. Abrams and the University of California to undertake the revised study, which began in December of 1997.[23] While this new version of the Abrams' study is designed to determine how cannabinoid use affects the use of protease inhibitors, and is specifically not a test of marijuana's medical utility, Dr. Abrams is committed to collecting a wealth of data on the effectiveness of marijuana in use by AIDS patients.[24]

The National Institutes of Health has officially recognized the medical utility of marijuana in combating the AIDS epidemic,[25] and the Institute of Medicine (IOM) has reported that marijuana is effective in fighting the many symptoms of wasting syndrome. The Executive Summary of the groundbreaking IOM report includes this detailed endorsement in a list of therapeutic effects:

> Third, for cases that are multifaceted, the combination of THC effects might provide a form of adjunctive therapy; for example, AIDS wasting patients would likely benefit from a medication that simultaneously reduces anxiety, pain, and nausea while stimulating appetite.[26]

On one hand, Drug Czar McCaffrey has signaled a lack of support for these recommendations,[27] and federal approval of FDA research that might lead to legalization of cannabis for medical uses seems unlikely.[28] Following the release of the IOM's *Marijuana and Medicine: Assessing the Science Base*, the Clinton administration did announce a policy reversal, saying it would loosen restrictions on marijuana research as early as December 1999.[29] Nonetheless, informed observers remain unconvinced, reminding us that legitimate studies on cannabis designed by state legislatures, universities, and private researchers have been repeatedly denied for more than 22 years. Chuck Thomas of the Marijuana Policy Project has criticized the continued stall tactics: "The Institute of Medicine recommended legal access for patients who need marijuana now, but the Clinton Administration rejected this recommendation. In effect, the Clinton Administration is therefore supporting the continued criminalization of these patients while the research drags on."

At whatever pace the government will allow, cannabinoid research is unlikely to deter America's war on marijuana in the foreseeable future. As Donald Abrams, the one scientist yet allowed to conduct a government-approved study on medical marijuana, has learned, only tests of safety are acceptable. Clinical studies that are designed to measure the effectiveness of marijuana as medicine will probably not be allowed because those studies might be applicable as evidence for FDA approval of the natural medicinal resource.[30] In all probability, the IOM recommendations on marijuana in medical trials will serve only those pharmaceutical companies that are willing to invest millions of dollars developing patented forms of synthetic cannabinoids.

While the federal government continues to block the legalization of medical marijuana, experts in the field are increasingly convinced of its value. The American Medical Association is only one of the many medical authorities that has urged the National Institutes of Health to support further studies.[31] Other medical and political groups have called for immediate access to the herbal medication, regardless of FDA approval. Organizations and groups (such as the seventeen most prominent AIDS coalitions, the AIDS Treatment News, the American Academy of Family Physicians, the American Medical Student Association, at least 44% of American oncologists,[32] the American Preventative Medical Association, the American Public Health Association, the American Society of Addictive Medicine, the British Medical Association,[33] the California Medical Association,[34] the California Society on Addiction Medicine, the Florida Medical Association, the Los Angeles County AIDS Commission, the Lymphoma Foundation of America, the Maine AIDS Alliance, the Marin Medical Society, the National Nurses Society on Addictions, *The New England Journal of Medicine*, the New Mexico State Board of Nursing, the Chairman of the New York State Assembly Committee on Health,[35] the North Carolina Nurses Association, the Oakland City Counsel,[36] the Royal College of

Physicians,[37] the Royal Pharmaceutical Society (UK),[38] the San Francisco Mayor's Office, the San Francisco Medical Society, the Virginia Nurses Association, 70% of all physicians in the United Kingdom[39]), and a majority of American citizens in statewide ballot initiatives and have all voiced support for legalizing the use of medical cannabis immediately, regardless of further studies.[40]

In the opening remarks at the Institute of Medicine's news conference on Marijuana and Medicine, Principal Investigator John Benson seemed to echo a similar sentiment: "[W]e concluded that there are some limited circumstances in which we recommend smoking marijuana for medical uses."[41] Seven months later, In *U.S. v. Oakland Cannabis Buyer's Club*, a three judge panel of the 9th U.S. Circuit Court of Appeals unanimously ruled:

> [T]here is a class of people with serious medical conditions
> for whom the use of cannabis is necessary in order to treat
> or alleviate those conditions or their symptoms; who will
> suffer serious harm if they are denied cannabis; and for
> whom there is no legal alternative to cannabis for the
> effective treatment of their medical conditions because
> they have tried other alternatives and have found that
> they are ineffective, or that they result in intolerable
> side effects.[42]

While that landmark federal ruling clearly recognized the medical necessity of marijuana use for victims of the AIDS epidemic, it was soon challenged by the Department of Justice. A humane resolution to this clash between law and medicine appears as elusive as the discovery of a cure for the deadly disease.

Related sections: *Cancer*, page 42; *Digestive Disorders* page 61; *Immune Responses*, page 70; *Marinol*, page 76; *Replacement of Medications*, page 97; *Smoking Methods*, page 107; *Stress Reduction*, page 109.

Addiction

Addiction is generally defined as physical or psychological dependence on a substance, especially alcohol or other drugs, with use of increasing amounts.[1] For the sake of clarification, this book defines physical addiction separately from psychological dependence. (See also the section entitled *Dependence*.) Scientific research on cannabinoid compounds has not demonstrated a strong association with biochemical addiction. In their exhaustive quest for evidence of addiction, federally funded researchers have resorted to relying on questionable data, such as the withdrawal symptoms reported by children who were referred to social service and criminal justice agencies. These researchers may argue that the court-ordered testimony of troubled youths "proves" that marijuana is addictive;[2] however, such questionable data is not scientific evidence of chemical addiction. In another case, an addictions researcher reported on his experiment in which rats displayed withdrawal symptoms upon a sudden discontinuation of THC. Critics point out that the reported withdrawal effects were created with very high doses of THC, and by the introduction of a second drug, a THC-blocking agent used to trigger the withdrawal symptoms. Withdrawal symptoms are not found in rats without using a THC-blocking agent,[3] and even among troubled youths, withdrawal symptoms are relatively mild and of short duration.[4,5]

Dopamine, a neurochemical produced in the central cortex of the brain, is thought to provide the brain's "reward system." Interference with dopamine production is considered a major symptom of biochemical addiction. While two studies alleged a minor link between THC and dopamine production in the brains of rats,[6] these were refuted by several subsequent studies showing that cannabis does not radically affect dopamine levels.[7,8,9] In assessing the importance of a possible link between cannabis use and dopamine levels, it should be noted that dopamine activity has also been detected in the brains of video game players who were paid money every time they reached a new level of the game.[10] Clearly, minor evidence of dopamine activity is not the sole indicator of addiction. If it were, then all pleasurable activities would be defined as addictive. Moreover, the scientific evidence that cannabis use produces any amount of increased dopamine activity remains entirely inconclusive. Assessing the scientific literature on marijuana's addictive potential for the Criminal Justice Commission of Australia, Peter Nelson reported, ". . . involvement with the ventromedial striatum suggests connections to dopamine circuits. However, the expected reinforcing properties usually associated with these dopamine pathways are difficult to demonstrate in the case of THC."[11]

Cannabinoids bond to anandamide nerve receptors that are primarily concentrated in the frontal lobes of the brain,[12,13] rather than the central cortex where dopamine is produced. THC is mild, with effects resembling those of caffeine or chocolate rather than classic addictive drugs such as alcohol, amphetamines, cocaine, opiates, and nicotine. In fact, a 1996 report from Daniele Piomelli of the Neurosciences Institute in San Diego indicated that chocolate contains three compounds that are chemically similar to cannabinoids. Studies involving rats showed that cannabinoid chemicals found in chocolate amplify the effect of natural cannabinoids found in the brain. The article published in *Nature* concluded that these compounds may "participate in the subjective feelings of eating chocolate."[14] In the April 1999 issue of *Nature Neuroscience*, Piomelli and colleagues at the University of California, Irvine reported that anandamide acts as an inhibitor of dopaminergic neurons.[15] Far from triggering chemical addiction in the brain, THC, the natural anandamide analogue, may actually help to balance erratic dopamine levels.

The common scientific criteria for determining the addictive quality of a drug are examples of animal studies in which subjects self-administer an addictive substance. When given the choice between food and narcotics, for example, animals commonly self-administer the drug to the exclusion of all other activity, often starving themselves to death. Unlike heroin, cocaine, and other substances of abuse, there are no clinical studies showing animals self-administering cannabinoid compounds. In 1993, the Congressional Office of Technology Assessment reached this conclusion:

> While marijuana produces a feeling of euphoria in humans, in general, animals will not self-administer THC in controlled studies. Also, cannabinoids generally do not lower the threshold needed to get animals to self-stimulate the brain reward system, as do other drugs of abuse.[16]

Clinical studies indicate a very low potential for addiction to cannabinoid drugs. In addition, there is no real-world evidence suggesting that THC is chemically addictive.[17] Epidemiological studies show that the large majority of people who try marijuana do not continue to use it on a regular basis. Moreover, the majority of those who ever use cannabis stop using it entirely before the age of thirty. Of an estimated 65 million "experimenters,"[18] only about 0.8% of Americans use cannabis on a daily basis.[19] The fact that millions of Americans have stopped using marijuana voluntarily and without difficulty is strong epidemiological evidence that cannabis is not chemically addictive.

Despite federally funded sociological and scientific findings that marijuana produces only mild dependence in some heavy users,[20,21] the federal government has officially classified cannabis as a Schedule I substance that has "a high potential for abuse." Recent research determining that cannabinoids are not chemically addictive and do not have a high potential for abuse forms the basis of a petition filed with the Drug Enforcement Administration. That petition prompted the federal drug agency to enter into a legally binding review of the existent evidence by the US Department of Health and Human Services in 1997.[22] Two years later, investigative authors of the 1999 Institute of Medicine report determined that ". . . marijuana was not particularly addictive."[23] Yet cannabis is still classified as having "no medical value and a high potential for abuse." In 1999, Dr. Podrebarac wrote to the White House Office of National Drug Control Policy: "The recently released Institute of Medicine (IOM) study on the medical use of marijuana clearly supports rescheduling it for medical use." The US Drug Czar's office refused to comment on the rescheduling issue. (See *Appendix*.)

Related sections: *Cerebral Effects*, page 49; *Dependence*, page 57; *Tolerance*, page 113; *Treating Addiction*, page 115.

Analgesia

Analgesia is the medical term for pain relief. Recent medical research emphasizes the need for increased treatment of chronic and incurable pain. New models of pain clarify understanding and thereby promote compassion. We now know that injured tissue sprouts new nerve fibers with even greater sensitivity to pain, a condition known as hyperalgia.[1] This increased level of sensitivity to pain after injury is a natural biological response that cannot be ignored. Sadly, the complaints of ill and aged people all too often go unanswered. A recent study of elderly cancer patients in nursing homes discovered that many cases are severely under-treated for pain relief. Of 4,003 cases studied, 26% received no pain medication at all, not even aspirin.[2] A similar 1998 finding that as many as

50% of all pain cases are under-treated prompted American medical experts to call for a "war on pain" with greater use of opiate painkillers.[3] In 1998, the *Journal of the American Medical Association* concluded that under-treatment of pain "is no longer acceptable and should be considered a first-line indicator of poor quality medical care."[4] The US Drug Enforcement Administration (DEA) is also in support of the new "war on pain," actively endorsing and encouraging the use of "in particular, narcotic analgesics [that] may be used in the treatment of pain experienced by a patient with a terminal illness or chronic disorder."[5] Unfortunately, analgesic drugs endorsed by the DEA have some seriously adverse effects, including headaches, nausea, addiction, loss of coordination, deep sedation, severe gastrointestinal disturbances, liver disease, kidney disease, and death. In fact, as *The New England Journal of Medicine* points out:

> It is also hypocritical to forbid physicians to prescribe marijuana while permitting them to use morphine and meperidine [Demerol], to relieve extreme dyspnea [shortness of breath] and pain. With both these drugs the difference between the dose that relieves symptoms and the dose that hastens death is very narrow; by contrast, there is no risk of death from smoking marijuana.[6]

The greater share of historical references to cannabis in medicine generally describe its analgesic actions. Specific citations on pain relief are common in most antiquated medical texts.[7,8] Modern research has verified those historical observations. Cannabinoids are effective in treating intractable (incurable) pain caused by a variety of conditions. In 1974, noted researchers Noyes and Baram studied five case histories and concluded, "There are indications that the active ingredient in marijuana may be a mild, though effective analgesic that is efficacious in functional pain."[9]

Besides THC, cannabis is known to contain several other effective cannabinoid and noncannabinoid compounds that

ANALGESIA

reduce painful inflammation.[10] A 1988 study found that cannabidiol, a cannabinoid not found in Marinol tablets, was more effective than aspirin in reducing inflammation.[11] Another paper, entitled "Delta-9-tetrahydrocannabinol Shows Antispastic And Analgesic Effects In A Single Case Double-Blind Trial," reached a similar conclusion.[12] Also in 1988, research by the University of London School of Pharmacy indicated that cannabinoids are not only effective pain relievers but would also be useful in the treatment of certain inflammatory disorders.[13]

Ten years later, a new model of pain relief has taken cannabinoid research to its next frontier. Atlantic Pharmaceuticals recently announced that it was evaluating the medical potential of a nonpsychoactive cannabinoid derivative of THC called CT-3. The company reported, "In recent studies, the agent was found to reduce inflammation and prevent destruction of joint tissue."[14]

Many other cannabinoids are also receiving attention for their great potential to reduce pain. In November 1997, Dr. Ian Meng reported to the public on research he had recently presented at the Society for Neuroscience meeting in October, "A synthetic marijuana-like drug called WIN 55212 enhances the brain's ability to suppress pain in rats, and probably in humans as well." In an interview on the subject, Meng elucidated the findings of his research team:

> People know that they [cannabinoids] are analgesic. But until fairly recently it hasn't been proven in animal studies that cannabinoids affect sensation.... I can actually look at the electrical impulses that travel down neurons to tell me how active a cell is. By doing that we've been able to show it's not just motor effects; this cannabinoid has very specific sensory effects. It affects the neurons in the pain pathway.[15]

The powerful opiate morphine replaced cannabis for the treatment of pain in the late 1800s, but now, 100 years later, modern research promises to reinstate cannabinoids as the premiere relievers of physical pain. In that same 1997 Society for Neuroscience conference, researchers from eight respected universities, Wake Forest University Medical School, the University of Michigan Medical School, the University of California at San Francisco (Meng et al.), Brown University, the University of Minnesota, and the University of Texas, each presented their individual evidence demonstrating that cannabinoids have a direct effect on biochemical pain signals in the central nervous system. Scientists reported that these cannabinoid studies reveal the potential for a new class of pain-control drugs superior to addictive opiate-based narcotics. Cannabinoids were shown to reduce pain through the central nervous system and also prevent the condition of hyperalgia, increased sensitivity to pain caused by injury. Scientists believe, therefore, that cannabinoids may be particularly effective in the treatment of arthritic pain.[16,17]

Researchers at the Medical College of Virginia reported that the presence of cannabinoid binding sites in the nervous system indicates that naturally occurring cannabinoids may govern the body's basic threshold of pain.[18] Research by the American Association for the Advancement of Science has produced similar findings.[19] Some scientists believe that cannabis is a more effective painkiller than opiates because the number of cannabinoid receptor sites found in the spinal cord is 10 to 50 times greater than the number of opiate receptors.[20]

A 1998 Nature article detailed how anandamide receptors located outside the central nervous system are crucial to pain control in cases of injury.[21] Also in 1998, studies at UCSF by Meng et al. showed that THC and morphine both affect the same cranial nerves located at the base of the skull. These studies were the first published evidence that cannabis has analgesic actions that work directly on the brain.[22]

When interviewed on cannabinoid analgesia, Dr. Ken Mackie, Professor of Anesthesiology at the University of Washington, replied, "Yes, marijuana does ease pain. As an analgesic it is about as efficacious as codeine."[23] Dr. Donald Abrams, Director of HIV Research at San Francisco General Hospital, explained why cannabis is actually superior to many common pharmeceutical painkillers:

> Cannabinoid-induced analgesia appears linked to the same system by which opioids [synthetic narcotics] produce pain relief. But different from opioids, cannabinoids are also effective in a rat model of neuropathic pain, which means pain caused by nerves. For those of us that care for people with HIV—we know about the painful, peripheral neuropathy they get—very painful, numb, tingling feet. We often start these patients on a trail of drugs that lead ultimately to morphine, because there isn't anything effective.[24]

A research paper done at Hammersmith Hospital in London confirmed cannabis' analgesic effects in the first UK clinical trial. The paper's abstract began, "Cannabinoids have analgesic and, possibly, anti-inflammatory properties but their clinical use has been restricted by legislation." That same abstract calling for further studies concluded, "Cannabis naïve patients would tolerate investigations but may generate medicolegal problems."[25]

The use of cannabis for pain relief was widespread in the membership of legitimate medical marijuana groups under attack by the US government.[26] In 1998, federal law enforcers closed San Francisco Bay Area Cannabis Clubs, forcing over 10,000 seriously ill patients to support nefarious "street" sources and pay outrageous black market prices for nonmedical grade marijuana. In the following year, the government-sponsored Institute of Medicine report elevated pain relief to the top of the list of marijuana's medical benefits.[27]

Related sections: *Addiction*, page 29; *Arthritis*, page 40; *Neuralgia*, page 85; *Psychoactivity*, page 91; *Replacement of Medications*, page 97.

Anorexia

Anorexia is an acute loss of appetite, often associated with psychological factors. Various stomach disorders, reactions to medications, and the use of illicit narcotics such as cocaine or heroin can cause anorexia. Some forms are thought to develop as an exaggerated response to cultural standards of beauty. While the relief of anorexia with the use of cannabis in those cases may also be related to psychological factors, the overwhelming evidence of the hunger-inducing properties of cannabinoids, particularly the primary ingredient, delta-9 THC, is current medical fact. Synthetic THC pills called Marinol are indicated for the treatment of anorexia, but physicians may risk losing their license by writing "off-label" Marinol prescriptions for patients suffering from anorexia not caused by the AIDS wasting syndrome or cancer chemotherapy.

Related sections: *AIDS*, page 21; *Digestive Disorders*, page 61; *Psychoactivity*, page 91; *Stress Reduction*, page 109.

Antibiotic Properties

Antibiotic Properties of cannabis extracts applied to the surface of an infected area have been reported in both historical and modern times. Cannabinoids can kill bacteria that have proven resistant to commonly used antibiotics. In one documented case a researcher inadvertently injured his thumb during a dissection. The penicillin resistant infection became so severe that amputation seemed the only reasonable option. Amputation was unnecessary, however, because the infection was finally overcome with topical application of cannabidolic acid.[1]

Antimotivational Syndrome

Antimotivational Syndrome has been one of the major premises of prohibitionist arguments. Cannabis is said to create an indifferent and apathetic attitude. This premise is completely unfounded. According to the UN World Health Organization in 1997, "The evidence for an antimotivational syndrome consists largely of case histories and observational reports."[1] Controlled studies have not found compelling evidence for such a syndrome.[2,3] The National Academy of Sciences noted that, "Over the past forty years, marijuana has been accused of causing an array of anti-social effects, including . . . destroying the American work ethic in young people. [These] beliefs . . . have not been substantiated by scientific evidence."[4]

Cases offered as proof that marijuana causes a loss of ambition may actually show that a lack of enthusiasm and psychological dependence on cannabis are both caused by an underlying depression. Moreover, in a highly competitive society, the development of alternative attitudes and values may easily be misinterpreted as antimotivational behavior.

In contrast to US prohibition rhetoric, Jamaican and Costa Rican studies report that field workers smoke marijuana during work in order to boost productivity.[5] In addition, studies of American college students have failed to establish evidence of an amotivational syndrome linked to cannabis use. One study of college students reported that users were found to have higher grades than nonusers, and another study reported that marijuana users scored higher than nonusers on standardized achievement scales.

Neuropsychological testing has failed to establish evidence of amotivational cerebral functions in studies involving a cannabis-consuming religious sect that showed no amotivational syndrome and no impairment of cognitive functions.[6]

Related sections: *Cerebral Effects*, page 49; *Depression*, page 59; *Psychoactivity*, page 91; *Tolerance*, page 113.

Anxiety Attacks

Anxiety Attacks have been reported among some novice cannabis users and also among some Marinol recipients. Three primary causes are cited: 1) Some clinical studies have relied on cannabis obtained "on the street" and consumed by persons having no prior experience with the illegal drug, generating a certain amount of anxiety, which seems appropriate, and is therefore easily discounted; 2) Novice users may simply be unaccustomed to the effects of cannabis, and therefore may in some cases interpret a slight increase in their circulation and heart rate as feelings of anxiety; 3) Synthetic delta-9 THC is known to be much more psychoactive than other cannabinoids present in natural marijuana, and is more potent than natural cannabis. At least one of the cannabinoids not found in Marinol, CBG, is known to have a sedative and anticonvulsant effect that counters the mental stimulation of THC.

Whatever the cause of anxiety attacks reported by a few users, such feelings are easily calmed by reassurance. Anxiety attacks generally subside in several minutes as the psychotropic effects dissipate.

Related sections: *Cardiovascular Effects*, page 47; *Incarceration*, page 72; *Paranoia Attacks*, page 90; *Psychoactivity*, page 91.

Arthritis

Arthritis is the inflammation of a joint accompanied by pain and swelling. An estimated 97 million Americans suffer from severe arthritis.[1] Relieving swelling and inflammation is one of the oldest recorded uses of cannabis. Modern science is currently exploring a newly discovered network of cannabinoid receptor sites located throughout the body. The new understandings of cannabinoid research clearly support historical references on treating inflammation with marijuana.

While synthetic THC has been found beneficial as an analgesic, clinical studies indicate that several other cannabinoids have more effective anti-inflammatory properties. Nonpsychoactive cannabis compounds such as CBD and CBG have greater anti-inflammatory properties than the legal THC pill.[2] One prominent researcher reported that CBC, a nonpsychoactive cannabinoid found abundant in certain strains of African cannabis, and some non-cannabinoid constituents of cannabis, olivitol, and cannoflavin, all have marked anti-inflammatory properties.[3]

In 1997, Kenneth Hargreaves of the University of Texas reported on research he conducted while at the University of Minnesota. In his words, "These results suggest that local administration of the cannabinoid to the site of injury may be able to both prevent pain from occurring and reduce pain which has already occurred without producing side-effects."[4] The Institute of Medicine report of 1999 recommends further study of these cannabinoids: "Because different cannabinoids appear to have different effects, cannabinoid research should include, but not be restricted to, effects attributable to THC alone."[5] Despite these promising recommendations, political and economic considerations rule the pharmaceutical marketplace. At the present time, marijuana remains the only available source of these naturally occurring anti-inflammatory compounds.

Related sections: *Analgesia*, page 32; *Replacement of Medications*, page 97.

Asthma

Asthma is the shortness of breath and wheezing caused by spasms of the bronchial tubes, overproduction of mucus, and swelling of the mucous membranes. Asthma kills more than 4,000 Americans each year.[1]

Clinical research shows that THC acts as a bronchial dilator, clearing blocked air passageways and allowing free breathing.[2,3] In one study, marijuana "caused an immediate reversal of exercise-induced asthma and hyperinflation."[4] Numerous cases of asthma have been treated successfully with both natural and synthetic THC.[5] In one report, a young woman used marijuana with her doctor's approval. Over the course of several years her attacks were almost completely cured with low doses of inhaled cannabis smoke.[6]

Some asthmatics who have found relief through the use of synthetic THC often voice a preference for natural cannabis over Marinol. Marinol is said to be less effective than natural cannabis and has far greater psychoactive properties.

Alternative methods of administration have been recommended by the Institute of Medicine[7] and other medical authorities. Plans for a noncombusting THC inhaler received attention for many years, yet designers have failed to produce a workable prototype.[8]

Related sections: *Immune Responses*, page 70; *Muscle Spasms*, page 83; *Psychoactivity*, page 91; *Respiratory Disease*, page 101; *Smoking Methods*, page 107; *Stress Reduction*, page 109

Cancer

Cancer is a broad term that refers to a wide range of cellular diseases typified by the abnormal development of a group of cells. The aberrant tendencies of these abnormal cells eventually disable the host organs. Cancerous cells are continually created in the body, but natural defenses usually counteract the disorganized cellular development in its incipient stages. Specific irritants, called carcinogens, may antagonize natural defenses, leading to the continued development of renegade cells. Unchecked, these outlaw cells frequently spread to surrounding tissue and may enter the lymphatic and circulatory systems, thereby spreading to other parts of the body. Removal of cancerous tissue by surgery and destruction of cancerous tissue by powerful chemotherapy and radiation therapy are the most common medical treatments.

Radiation and chemotherapy often induce violent, gut-wrenching nausea. Delta-9 THC is legally prescribed for counteracting the severe side effects of these cancer therapies, and is prescribed by doctors under its trade name, Marinol. Marinol pills, which are taken orally to control vomiting, were shown to be a superior antiemetic (antinausea drug) in six out of seven well-controlled studies reported in the *Journal of the*

American Medical Association as early as 1981.[1] In earlier scientific studies, Marinol was also proven superior to other antiemetics.[2,3] However, Marinol falls short of perfection because of its super high potency, which often leads to intoxication and sedation.[4,5] Also, oral administration is the least preferable method in this circumstance.

The paradox of swallowing a pill to eliminate vomiting has been noted by many physicians and patients, as well as the American Medical Association.[6] Ralph Seeley, an attorney who petitioned the State of Washington for access to medical cannabis and later died of bone cancer, was quick to point out, "I don't know how many times I've taken one of those $12 pills and had it come right back up."[7] Marijuana is commonly smoked, which is a quicker and more effective method than oral administration. In the words of the National Cancer Institute, "Marijuana cigarettes have been used to treat chemotherapy-induced nausea and vomiting, and research has shown that THC is more quickly absorbed from marijuana smoke than from an oral preparation."[8]

A careful study determining that marijuana is more effective than Marinol was published in 1988,[9] but only one other research group, the Tennessee Board of Pharmacy, has been bold enough to confirm those findings.[10] The National Institutes of Health is officially knowledgeable that smoked marijuana is more effective than Marinol tablets; panelists of the NIH Workshop on the Medical Utility of Marijuana in 1997 made very strong statements about marijuana's safety and medical value.[11] However, the National Institute on Drug Abuse, sole source of federal cannabis for legal research, does not support scientific investigations that might lead to rescheduling marijuana as medicine. As Donald Abrams, the one researcher allowed to study smoked cannabis, has discovered, clinical trials on marijuana as medicine may be approved as tests for medical safety only, not as tests for medical effectiveness.[12]

Marinol, the antiemetic "rescue drug," is directed for prescription when other medications fail, but research indicates that delta-9 THC is not the only cannabis constituent worthy of medical administration to relieve vomiting. A report from the Brettler Center for Medical Research at Hebrew University in Jerusalem administered delta-8 THC, a nonpsychoactive cannabinoid not found in the Marinol tablet, to eight children receiving chemotherapy treatments. Reportedly, "Vomiting was completely prevented."[13] It is clear that the Marinol pill does not contain the complete range of medicinal cannabinoids shown to be effective in treating severe nausea.

Many patients agree that Marinol is less effective than whole marijuana, and many cancer specialists concur. In 1991, 44% of oncologists surveyed said they had already recommended cannabis to their patients, and 56% said that marijuana should be legally prescribable.[14] As early as 1975 the *New England Journal of Medicine* had reported that "THC is an effective antiemetic for patients receiving cancer chemotherapy."[15] Since then, dozens of scientific studies recognized by the US Food and Drug Administration and the National Cancer Institute have shown that the use of natural cannabis is a preferable remedy for adverse effects of the cancer-killing poisons employed in oncology.[16] Relief from the side effects of cancer chemotherapy is a widely accepted medical use of marijuana in the United States. The American Cancer Society is one of dozens of national and international health organizations that have voiced support for further research on the medical use of cannabis in cancer chemotherapy treatments.[17]

In addition to its well known antinausea effects, marijuana often relieves physical pain associated with cancer,[18] a finding that is supported by published research studies,[19] the testimony of physicians,[20] and the reports of the Institute of Medicine (IOM).[21] Some cancer survivors even claim that continued use of cannabis helps keep their disease in remission—a possibility that cannot be discounted in light of research by the National Toxicology Program.

Independent studies in the mid-1970s suggested that cannabinoids inhibited tumor growth in lab mice.[22] In 1979, a study commissioned by the Australian government concluded that cannabis is effective in the treatment of glaucoma, and "of potentially greater significance is the recent finding that THC inhibits the growth of some types of cancer in tissue culture."[23] Intriguing as they may be, those citations pale in light of investigations by the US government. Ironically, pursuing common prohibitionist rhetoric proved quite perplexing upon analyzing the carcinogenic properties of THC. In the mid-1990s, the US federal government funded a two-year and two-million-dollar study by the National Toxicology Program under the review of the Federal Drug Administration, the National Cancer Institute, and other federal agencies. The study was designed to determine the cancer rate induced by injecting high doses of THC into the bodies of mice, then injecting them with cancerous cells. Ironically, the study found that the mice injected with THC had a far lower incidence of cancer than did the control group. Assessing the unpublished draft version, cannabis researcher Donald Abrams summarized, "THC caused fewer tumors and prolonged survival in these laboratory animals."[24] The deputy director of the National Toxicology Program study concurred, "We found absolutely no evidence of cancer." The profound implication that cannabis use might actually help prevent cancer has not been officially released to the American public, purportedly because of a lack of personnel.[25,26] The executive secretary of the Toxicology Program study has remarked, "I think it's terrible the way the government is handling this marijuana issue. There's no reason this shouldn't have been published."[27]

Even without the Toxicology Program study, some leading scientists were already aware of this remarkable potential. Marijuana researcher Leo Hollister has noted the apparent dichotomy of investigations on cannabis and cancer:

The clinical implication of some of these findings is obscure. On the one hand, exposure to smoke from cannabis may be carcinogenic. On the other, the changes in nucleic acid synthesis, were they to be specific for rapidly dividing cells, such as those of malignancies, might be useful therapeutically in their treatment.[28]

The Institute of Medicine report of 1999 failed to address this intriguing potential of cannabinoid medicines in the prevention and treatment of cancer because the National Toxicology Program study had not been officially published. Instead, the popular subject of respiratory cancer figured heavily in the million-dollar report commissioned by the White House Office of National Drug Control Policy. However, the IOM Executive Summary cautiously avoided drawing negative conclusions from the available data:

> Although cellular, genetic, and human studies all suggest that marijuana smoke is an important risk factor for the development of respiratory cancer, proof that habitual marijuana smoking does or does not cause cancer awaits the results of well-designed studies.[29]

For generations, prohibitionists have argued that smoking cannabis causes cancer, yet the government's own National Toxicology Program study indicated that cannabis might actually help prevent cancer. After reviewing sixteen years of government studies on cannabis and respiratory cancer, the IOM report cites a lack of proof and calls for even more research. In the words of Stanford researcher Leo Hollister, "If field studies fail to provide evidence of harm from prolonged use of cannabis, it is unlikely that experimental studies will do better, and such has been the case." [30]

Related sections: *AIDS*, page 21; *Anorexia*, page 37; *Analgesia*, page 32; *Marinol*, page 76; *Respiratory Disease*, page 101.

Cardiovascular Effects

Cardiovascular Effects on the heart and blood vessels are marked by a 20% to 50% increase in the heart rate and a mild decrease in blood pressure, though the documented effects of cannabis on fluid blood pressure are inconsistent. Pressure within the blood vessels appears to decrease mildly with continued use (mild hypotension), but some research has shown the opposite effect (mild hypertension).[1] The heart rate (beats per minute) increases slightly for up to 30 minutes following smoked inhalation and longer for oral ingestion. These effects subside over the following 2 to 4 hours. In chronic long-term use, a slightly depressed heart rate and slight lowering of blood pressure (hypotension) has been observed.[2]

These distinct cardiovascular effects of cannabinoids have been the focus of many debates among scientists. Peter Nelson, in the employ of the Criminal Justice System of Australia, noted the subjective nature of certain researchers' scientific evaluations:

> Jones claims that THC has "far more effect (on the cardiovascular system) than nicotine," but fails to tell us how. In fact, the findings of Benowitz and Jones he presents on long term oral administration of THC (above) shows an effect which could be construed as potentially useful in combating the negative cardiovascular effects of long term stress. As is often the case in THC research, interpretation is in the eye of the beholder.[3]

CARDIOVASCULAR EFFECTS

Nelson also informed the Australian government that, "His [Jones'] statements comparing nicotine with THC are particularly ill founded."[4]

In a 1979 paper titled, *Effect of marijuana on cardiorespiratory responses to submaximal exercise*, it was reported that

> Smoking [marijuana] had no effect on blood pressure, pulmonary ventilation and oxygen uptake, but did include a marked increase in heart rate which persisted throughout exercise and recovery periods, averaging 34% higher than control values at rest, 18% higher during exercise, and up to 50% higher during recovery.[5]

In 1997, the United Nations World Health Organization report found no cause for alarm:

> The conclusion reached by the Institute of Medicine in 1982 still stands: the smoking of marijuana causes changes to the heart and circulation that are characteristic of stress.. .[but] there is no evidence ... that it exerts a permanently deleterious effect on the normal cardiovascular system.[6]

There is no reason to suspect that a slight increase of heartbeats per minute caused by cannabis use is any more injurious to the heart or other organs than normal physical exercise. A small increase in the heart rate may be considered beneficial to the entire body in allowing greater blood flow. In contrast, long-term chronic use is usually associated with a slight decrease in the heart rate.[7] A review of research by the Australian National Drug Strategy revealed that "Tolerance to the cardiovascular effects develops within seven to ten days in persons receiving high daily doses . . . [of THC]."[8]

Both field studies and electrocardiographic research have failed to detect cardiac pathology caused by cannabis use.[9] However, as a precaution, patients suffering from acute cardiac disease, such as angina pectoris, are usually advised by their physician to abstain from using marijuana.

One other notable vascular effect of cannabis is typically displayed in the dilation of blood vessels, causing a reddening of the eyes. The cannabis-induced "red-eye" symptom represents a general increase in cerebral blood flow.[10] The mild effect is temporary and is not considered injurious.

Related sections: *Respiratory Effects*, page 101; *Tolerance*, page 113.

Cerebral Effects

Cerebral Effects of cannabis use, such as biochemical addiction and the potential for cerebral damage, have been studied at some length. Current advances have discredited earlier claims and offered new insights into natural cannabinoids found in the brain.

Interference with dopamine production is the chemical basis of addiction in the use of alcohol, amphetamines, cocaine, nicotine, opiate compounds, and other powerful addictive substances. Clinical studies show that cannabis is dissimilar to classic addictive drugs in that it does not significantly interfere with dopamine production in the "pleasure centers" of the brain, according to the Office of Technology Assessment after ten years of research.[1]

Although one Italian researcher has reported a minor increase in dopamine activity (DA levels) associated with THC administration,[2] follow-up studies at the Brookhaven National Laboratories disagree. Examining the effects of cannabis on dopamine activity in rats, the Brookhaven Medical Department determined that

> ... unlike a number of drugs of abuse, THC does not alter the activity of A10 DA neurons and that the previously reported THC-induced increase in brain DA levels is not due to its action on firing rate or pattern in A10 DA neurons.[3]

49

The 1988 discovery of the CB1 receptor, found abundant in the brain, and the 1992 discovery of the CB2 receptor found throughout the body, clearly distinguish cannabinoid compounds from other substances.[4] Cannabinoids bind to anandamide receptors in the frontal lobes of the brain, according to research published by the American Association for the Advancement of Science.[5] Researchers from the Duke University Medical Center in North Carolina agree:

> Behavioral manifestations of marijuana intoxication may be associated with increased functional activity of the brain especially in the frontal cortex...and regression analysis indicated it correlated most markedly with the right frontal region.[6]

Anandamide is a natural neurotransmitter found in the brain that binds to the same neuroreceptors as do cannabinoids.[7,8] Current research suggests that cannabinoids are very similar to anandamide, which regulates mood, memory, pain, movement, and appetite.[9] Although these recent findings are not thoroughly understood, it is clear that cannabis affects the brain in ways completely dissimilar to other drugs, in accordance with natural neurochemical pathways.

While medical science makes remarkable discoveries on the potential of cannabinoid "wonder drugs," political dogma stagnates in denial. One 20-year-old study continues to fuel claims that cannabis use causes cerebral damage. Two unwitting rhesus monkeys were exposed to 200 times the normal human dose of THC, administered through a constant cloud of smoke. Months later, the monkeys' brains were dissected. Researchers reported discovering minor brain damage. However, in a more recent study, rhesus monkeys exposed to the equivalent of 5 cannabis cigarettes per day for seven months, (what would be termed heavy chronic use in an adult human) showed no signs of cerebral abnormalities, discrediting claims attached to the older study.[10]

A 1988 study of rhesus monkeys showed that high doses of THC impairs visual recognition memory, but not discrimination learning, even at very high doses.[11] While clinical testing of human subjects indicates that cannabis use mildly interferes with short-term memory functions in novice users, long-term memory and learning skills are not affected. Minor short-term memory impairment induced by acute cannabis intoxication is temporary. Experienced users who have developed a tolerance to the psychoactive drug frequently display no signs of cerebral impairment while under the influence of cannabis. The natural development of a tolerance to the cerebral effects of cannabinoids is well established and was clearly recognized by the Institute of Medicine in 1999.[12]

During Britain's recent movement toward reform of marijuana laws, hundreds of doctors and scientists have supplied evidence to the government detailing the therapeutic value and nonaddictive properties of cannabis. Professor Colin Blakemore, chairman of the British Neuroscience Association, told the members of a 1997 conference, "Efforts to prove the damaging effects of cannabis have produced little evidence of any harm to the brain and central nervous system."[13]

Jack Fletcher of the University of Texas has been testing the mental skills of heavy long-term cannabis users in Costa Rica for the past 25 years. Studying those who have smoked in the range of ten joints per day for more than thirty years, Fletcher has detected only minor cognitive impairments that fall well within normal ranges. Brian Page, an anthropologist from the University of Miami who also took part in the study notes that "The effects are subtle and subclinical."[14]

According to a study published by the prestigious American Association for the Advancement of Science, cognition is definitely not impaired by the chronic use of cannabis. A battery of scientific tests, including the *Wechsler Adult Intelligence Scale*, the *Benton Visual Retention Test*, and the *Rey Auditory-Verbal Learning Test*, in conjunction with urine analysis by the enzyme immunoassay method, were used to determine that heavy, long-term cannabis users showed no cognitive impairment compared to standardized norms.[15]

Dr. John P. Morgan of the City University of New York has said, "There is no convincing evidence that heavy long term marijuana use impairs memory or other cognitive functions. During the past 30 years, researchers have found, at most, minor cognitive differences between chronic marijuana users and nonusers, and the result differ substantially from one study to another."[16]

The first extensive US study of long term cognitive performance in a large population group was published in the May 1st 1999 issue of the American Journal of Epidemiology. 1,318 participants, including long term marijuana smokers, were given standard cognitive tests, called Mini-Mental-State Examinations, over a 12 year period. The research team from Johns Hopkins Hospital in Baltimore detected no abnormal decline in thinking skills among marijuana users. The study determined that:

> There were no significant differences in cognitive decline between heavy users, light users, and nonusers of cannabis. There were also no male-female differences in cognitive decline in relation to cannabis use. The authors conclude that over long time periods, in persons under age 65 years, cognitive decline occurs in all age groups. This decline is closely associated with aging and educational level but does not appear to be associated with cannabis use.[17]

A similar finding is reported by the United Nations World Health Organization, "The weight of the available evidence suggests that even the long term heavy use of cannabis does not produce any severe or grossly debilitating impairment of cognitive function."[18]

Research from the US National Institute for Mental Health has indicated that THC and another cannabis compound, cannabidiol, actually protect the brain from cellular damage caused by stroke, blood clots, and head injury.[19, 20]

Related sections: *Addiction*, page 29; *Dependence*, page 57; *Psychoactivity*, page 91; *Stroke and Head Trauma*, page 110; *Tolerance*, page 113.

Chromosome Interference

Chromosome Interference due to administration of cannabinoids has been studied at some length. There is great uncertainty as to the clinical significance of existing test tube studies. Whereas Nahas, a researcher long known for his negative interpretations of cannabinoid research, concluded that "cannabinoids and marijuana may exert a weak mutagenic effect," a less biased researcher reviewing the same evidence gave an entirely different interpretation, noting that *in vivo* and *in vitro* exposure to purified cannabinoids or cannabis resin failed to increase the frequency of chromosomal damage or mutagenesis.[1]

Splitting hairs over inconclusive evidence of chromosome interference caused by excessive doses of cannabinoids may fuel some scientific careers, but conclusions resulting from such speculation is easily discounted. Test-tube methods of creating chromosome breaks with cannabinoids could be duplicated with aspirin, valium, and many other pharmaceutical drugs. Moreover, DNA samplings of large populations of heavy users in cannabis-friendly countries have failed to show any abnormalities in chromosome structure.

Hollister states that "virtually every drug that has ever been studied for dysmorphogenic effects [chromosome interference leading to birth defects] has been found to have them if the doses are high enough, if enough species are tested, or if treatment is prolonged."[2] Other scientists conclude that "the

53

few reports of teratogenicity in rodents and rabbits indicate that cannabinoids are, at most, weakly teratogenic in these species."[3] According to the United Nations World Health Organization report of 1997, "There is not a great deal of evidence that cannabis use can produce chromosomal or genetic abnormalities in either parent which could be transmitted to the offspring."[4]

Related sections: *Cancer*, page 42; *Immune Responses*, page 70.

Constipation

Constipation of intestinal reflexes may be alleviated by the antiemetic properties of cannabis and synthetic THC tablets. Relief of constipation was one of the original cannabis indications cited by Shen-Nung five thousand years ago. Virtually every historical medical reference since that time has included similar observations. In comparison, opiate narcotics commonly cause very severe constipation in continued use.

Related sections: *Digestive Disorders*, page 61.

Contaminants

Contaminants contained in natural cannabis continue to pose a health threat to patients who must obtain their medicine from unscrupulous illicit markets. The popular fear is that illegal marijuana might be intentionally saturated with other illegal drugs. This possibility is unlikely, because intentional contamination with other illegal substances would not be economically feasible for the typical drug dealer. Ignorant purchasers might be duped into buying oregano or some other material resembling marijuana, but such costly mistakes are rarely repeated. Several common contaminant hazards are of more serious concern to most medical marijuana users.

Harmful pesticides may be absorbed by the marijuana plant during cultivation and then enter the human body through administration. The health hazards of these noxious chemicals are sometimes included as label warnings, often advising the grower to wear gloves and avoid inhalation. Repeated exposure to unknown chemical poisons may build to toxic levels in a user's system. Even the most well-intentioned marijuana farmer may be an unwitting supplier of pesticide poisons.

The US government provides another contaminant risk in its spraying programs intended to stop the use of marijuana. Herbicides used to eradicate illegal crops have many known health hazards.[1] The United States government sprayed the herbicide Paraquat on marijuana crops in Mexico years ago, and in Hawaii more recently. Paraquat and other Drug War pesticides permeate vegetative growth and are definitely injurious to human health. Excessively yellow marijuana may be tainted with Paraquat that can cause serious lung damage. Government sources have assured us that this military surplus poison is no longer in use, yet there are many other noxious poisons routinely applied to outdoor marijuana plants. In 1998, the Drug Enforcement Administration released plans to spray another herbicide, Triclopyr, on wild hemp fields across America.[2] Typically, these widespread crop eradication programs are executed without adherence to environmental impact studies required by law.[3] Even more alarming, crop eradication programs outside the United States operate with no concern for environmental or public health issues. For example, the industrial weed killer, Tebuthiurin, is so strong that a few granules spread on grass tufts can kill trees located several yards away. Contamination of water supplies with Tebuthiurin could cause widespread destruction of entire ecosystems. Dow Chemical Corporation, manufacturer of the toxic defoliant called *Agent Orange* during the Vietnam War, is one of several corporations that sided with environmentalists in resisting a US plan to use Tebuthiurin in crop eradication programs in Colombia on an estimated 150,000 acres.[4] The intentional poisoning of rural landscapes by the government bodes ill for both the targeted outdoor marijuana gardens and for native wildlife. Drug eradication plans to unleash a new marijuana-eating fungus in America have met with harsh criticism. Bill Graves, senior biologist at the University of Florida Research Center, is concerned about the possibility of unpredictable mutations. Graves has said, "I believe that if this fungus is unleashed for this kind of problem, it's going to create its own problems. If it isn't executed effectively, it's going to target and kill rare and endangered species."[5] The effects of mutant bioherbicides on the health of medical marijuana consumers are unknown and impossible to predict.

A third contaminant hazard is found in bacterial or fungal infections produced by careless cultivation techniques. A majority of the several hundred organisms associated with marijuana are strictly plant pathogens that cannot infect humans. A smaller number of plant pathogens are also found in cannabis that has been improperly dried or stored. Some of these organisms may infect immune-suppressed individuals and become human pathogens. Also, a small handful of human pathogens have been isolated from samples of poor-quality marijuana. These contaminants are highly infectious and potentially toxic.[6]

Suppliers of medical grades of cannabis must be particularly stringent in their cultivation techniques because HIV and AIDS patients suffering from immune suppression typically comprise 75% of medical user populations. Properly cultivated marijuana and its constituent cannabinoid compounds are among the safest drugs known to medical science.[7,8,9]

Related sections: *Toxicity*, page 114.

Delirium

Delirium marked by memory impairment and disorientation has been observed in a few rare cases. These reports invariably originate in countries such as India where high-potency cannabis extracts are taken orally. Eating large quantities of high-potency marijuana, using concentrated cannabis called hashish, or taking multiple doses of synthetic delta-9 THC in tablet form is usually found to induce sedation and sleep. Delirium is uncommon, yet may appear in children and older people who are physiologically more susceptible to psychotropic drugs. Despite the few reported cases, there is no biochemical model for delirium caused by ingesting exceptionally large quantities of cannabinoid compounds. Reportedly, subjects suffering from cannabis-induced delirium are easily calmed by clear and rational discussion. All psychological and physiological effects of cannabis wear off within several hours following consumption.

Related sections: *Toxicity*, page 114.

Dependence

Dependence on marijuana by chronic, heavy users, or by persons predisposed to addictive behaviors is a potential development. Although psychological dependency can result in behaviors similar to those found in actual biochemical addiction, cannabis dependency rarely manifests in ways overtly harmful to the subject's life or lifestyle. Psychological dependence on any mind-altering substance may be caused by an underlying depression or by psychological turmoil. According to the Institute of Medicine (IOM), "Risk factors for marijuana dependence are similar to those for other forms of substance abuse."[1] However, those persons at risk for developing a psychological dependence to cannabinoids face a lesser threat than with other drugs. The IOM study also noted, "Animal research demonstrates the potential for dependence, but this potential is observed under a narrower range of conditions than with benzodiazepines [such as Valium], opiates, cocaine, or nicotine."[2]

Although epidemiological surveys show that cannabis dependence is the most common form of drug dependence due to its widespread availability, relatively few users voluntarily seek treatment for marijuana dependence, according to the American Psychiatric Association in 1994.[3] While a small percentage of the population may be prone to substance abuse, evidence suggests that the vast majority of marijuana users have discontinued their use on a voluntary basis.[4]

Patients who regularly use any medication may be labeled medically dependent on that medication's beneficial effects. Prohibitionists who reject the use of marijuana as a medicine may purposely misinterpret reasonable medical dependence as psychological dependence simply because cannabis is an illicit medication.

Related sections: *Addiction*, page 29; *Antimotivational Syndrome*, page 38; *Depression*, page 59.

Depression

Depression diagnosis by American physicians doubled in the 1990s, from 11 million to more than 20.4 million cases, according to the *Journal of the American Medical Association*.[1] Antidepressants such as Prozac now account for 45% of all prescribed psychoactive drugs. More than 130 million prescriptions were written for anti-depressant drugs in 1998. Yet, as in the case of Prozac, the benefits reported by patients are only marginally better than the result reported by patients given placebo drugs, according to studies observed by the FDA.[2] Psychiatrist Mikuriya cites dozens of historical and contemporary cases of the successful treatment of clinical depression with cannabis.[3] The antidepressant effects of marijuana have been confirmed in many human research studies.[4] Medically classified as a euphoriant, cannabis generally promotes nondepressive thoughts and feelings for most users.[5] Some people may naturally gravitate toward the use of marijuana for the relief of personal depression.[6] While chronic depression may lead to suicide, domestic violence, alcoholism, drug addiction, and other destructive behaviors, there are no similar health risks associated with the mild euphoria of marijuana intoxication.

Related sections: *Antimotivational Syndrome*, page 38; *Dependence*, page 57; *Psychoactivity*, page 91; *Stress Reduction*, page 109; *Tolerance*, page 113.

Diabetes

Diabetes is a condition wherein the body either produces inadequate amounts of insulin or fails to utilize available insulin properly. An estimated 1 million Americans suffer from type 1 diabetes, which develops in childhood. Another 15 million suffer from type 2 diabetes, which develops later in life.[1] Symptoms generally include an imbalance of blood sugar levels and a high level of sugar excreted through the urine. Initial studies showed that cannabis has no effect on blood sugar levels. A recent test-tube study showed that very high doses of synthetic THC might aggravate diabetes, but that same research also indicates that continued use of cannabis creates a tolerance to the potential aggravation.[2] No human studies have found that cannabis or synthetic cannabinoids contribute to symptoms of diabetes. At the same time, no human studies have been undertaken to prove or disprove the reports of long-term diabetics who claim that cannabis use causes an immediate lowering of abnormally high blood sugar levels.[3] Some diabetics also claim that cannabis helps stabilize blood sugar levels and maintain mental stability, or correct mood swings caused by fluctuating blood sugar levels.[4] Separating the apparent blood sugar response from the antianorexic properties of cannabis is currently a matter for further investigation.

Diabetics are frequently instructed to refrain from alcohol use because of its high caloric content. Cannabis may provide a psychologically valuable alternative to alcohol in stress reduction, a major factor in managing the potentially life-threatening symptoms of diabetes. Hence, cannabis may function in several ways to reduce and stabilize blood sugar levels for patients suffering from diabetes. However, regardless of mounting anecdotal evidence in medical practice, including medical testimony before a district court in California,[5] no scientific papers have been published on the effectiveness of cannabis in treating diabetes.

While cannabis has been used as a replacement for insulin, diabetics are strongly advised to continue their physician's prescribed treatment plan.

Related sections: *Insomnia*, page 75; *Psychoactivity*, page 91; *Stress Reduction*, page 109.

Digestive Disorders

Digestive Disorders, including anorexia, bulimia, the effects of cancer chemotherapy treatment, the AIDS wasting syndrome, intestinal diseases such as ileitis and colitis, spastic bowel, and morning sickness due to pregnancy all have diverse causes, but include common symptoms such as severe nausea and constipation, which are generally relieved by the use of cannabis.

The symptoms of ulcerative colitis were repeatedly relieved by smoked cannabis in a report published by the Annals of Internal Medicine in 1990.[1] Further research is limited, but anecdotal reports are plentiful.[2,3]

Related sections: *Constipation*, page 54; *Intestinal Cramps*, 75.

Dry Mouth

Dry Mouth is a common condition associated with inhalation of marijuana smoke, although research indicates that smoking methods are not the sole cause of this condition. Salivary flow is shown to be significantly decreased by oral administration

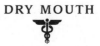

of Marinol, synthetic THC in pill form.[1] Water or other liquid beverages bring instant relief.

Related sections: *Tear Ducts*, page 112.

Dystonia

Dystonia is a prolonged involuntary muscle spasm that can occur in any muscle of the body. Dystonic conditions are often neurological in origin, but may also be caused by typical antipsychotic medications such as Thorazine. Cannabinoids are reported to be beneficial in controlling many types of spastic disorders. Medical experts in both America and Great Britain have expressed interest in further studies of cannabinoids in controlling spasticity.

Related sections: *Epilepsy*, page 62; *Huntington's Chorea*, page 68; *Multiple Sclerosis*, page 82; *Muscles Spasms*, page 83; *Neuralgia*, page 85.

Epilepsy

Epilepsy is a recurrent disorder of cerebral function characterized by sudden, brief attacks of altered consciousness, motor activity, or sensory phenomena. Epilepsy includes a broad range of seizure disorders caused by microscopic brain lesions occurring during birth or during traumatic head injury. Epileptics often lead normal lives that are sporadically interrupted by violent seizures.

Epilepsy is usually treated with barbiturates, benzodiazepines, and other powerful antiseizure medications that render the patient incapable of normal activity. Prescription anticonvulsants are not effective for 20-30% of epileptic patients. Many patients suffer intolerable, and sometimes fatal, complications from standard pharmaceutical medications. Some epileptics find that marijuana controls their seizures without causing the physical and psychological depression typical of pharmaceutical therapies.[1,2,3]

Animal studies indicate that several cannabinoids not found in the synthetic THC pill have notable anticonvulsant properties. For example CBD, one of many medicinal compounds not available by prescription, has been shown to completely control partial seizure disorders.[4] Marijuana is the only source of CBD and other cannabinoids that can help control the agony of epileptic attacks.

Recent US military tests reported that rats protected by synthetic cannabinoids were 70% less likely to suffer epileptic seizures and brain damage after exposure to nerve gas.[5]

Warning: epileptics should consult with their physician before using psychoactive drugs.

Related sections: *Cerebral Effects,* page 49; *Dystonia,* page 62; *Multiple Sclerosis,* page 82; *Muscle Spasms,* page 83; *Neuralgia,* page 85; *Psychoactivity,* page 91; *Replacement of Medications,* page 97; *Stroke and Head Trauma,* page 110.

Fertility

Fertility in both female and male humans is not significantly impaired by natural cannabis or isolated cannabinoid compounds. Animal studies have found that extremely high doses of synthetic THC can mildly inhibit ovulation and testosterone production, but that inhibition dissipated with continued administration. Some human studies show mild depression of hormone levels within normal basal ranges following administration of a large dose (2.0-2.8% THC cigarettes) of cannabis, but these levels also returned to normal upon continued exposure.[1] According to the Australian government's recent review of the available research data,

> Even if there are such effects of cannabis on male reproductive functioning, their clinical significance in humans is uncertain (Institute of Medicine, 1982) since testosterone levels in the studies which have found effects have generally remained within the normal range (Hollister, 1986) ... In the absence of any other human evidence, both Bloch (1983) and the Institute of Medicine (1982) argued on the basis of animal literature that cannabis use probably had an inhibitory effect on female reproductive function which was similar to that which occurs in males.[2]

Medical authorities Zimmer and Morgan offer real-world evidence and rational insight:

> There are no epidemiological studies showing that men who use marijuana have higher rates of infertility than men who do not. Nor is there evidence of diminished reproductive capacity among men in countries where marijuana use is common. It is possible that marijuana could cause infertility in men who already have low sperm counts. However, it is likely that regular marijuana users develop tolerance to marijuana's hormonal effects.[3]

Related sections: *Immune Responses*, page 70; *Obstetrics*, page 87; *Testosterone*, page 112; *Tolerance*, page 113.

Gateway

Gateway theories are among the most prevalent antimarijuana slogans. Prohibitionists contend that marijuana users graduate to stronger drugs. While it is true that the major portion of heroin users tried marijuana at some point in their life, it does not follow that every marijuana user will eventually become addicted to heroin. Surveys of narcotic abusers indicate that many did use marijuana before using harder drugs, but most also used other supposed gateway drugs, such as alcohol, tobacco, and caffeine, before trying marijuana. The vast majority of caffeine, tobacco, alcohol, or marijuana users do not advance to stronger drugs. Moreover, the majority of Americans who try marijuana (estimated in the tens of millions) do not continue to use cannabis on a habitual basis and often stop using it entirely by the age of 30. The 1999 Institute of Medicine report dismissed any previous credibility of the gateway theory, noting that tobacco and alcohol generally predate marijuana use as gateway drugs.

Related sections: *Addiction*, page 29; *Cerebral Effects*, page 49; *Dependence*, page 57.

Glaucoma

Glaucoma, the number two cause of blindness in the United States, is characterized by a dangerous increase of the fluid pressure within the eye. Glaucoma patient Robert Randall was the first person to receive federal approval for the use of cannabis after pioneering the medical necessity defense in Florida in 1976.[1] Although the American Academy of Opthalmology has strongly opposed the use of cannabis to treat glaucoma, the effectiveness of cannabis in relieving intraocular pressure has been demonstrated by numerous clinical trials, including those of the National Academy of Sciences. One study indicated that two cannabinoids, delta-8 THC and CBN, effectively reduced intraoccular pressure, but that two others, CBD, and delta-9 THC, the psychoactive ingredient of Marinol, did not.[2]

One major objection to cannabis use for the treatment of glaucoma is the apparent decrease in optic blood pressure associated with the decrease in intraocular fluid.[3] Another major objection is the relative duration of action. While cannabis is shown to be as effective at reducing intraocular pressure as other medications, the dose level must be maintained at three- or four-hour intervals, while other medications may be taken less frequently.

Scientists remain tantalized by the possibility of studying the effects of cannabinoids and of synthesizing more effective cannabinoid derivatives.[4] Although the medical application of cannabis is not endorsed by the American Society of Opthalmology[5] or the Institute of Medicine, and while the exact mechanism is not thoroughly understood, at least some physicians have the vision of Lester Grinspoon, M.D., who testified before Congress in 1997: "Cannabis does not cure the disease, but it can retard the progressive loss of sight when conventional medication fails and surgery is too dangerous."[6] Cannabinoid eye drops have decreased the ocular pressure of mice, but as yet have not been found effective in several human trials.[7,8,9] Related sections: *Psychoactivity*, page 91.

Hepatitis

Hepatitis is an inflammation of the liver caused by viral and toxic contaminants. Patients suffer painful enlargement of the liver and many other symptoms, including fever, chills, vomiting, severe jaundice, fatigue, and death. The deadly Hepatitis C Virus (HCV) accounts for 70% of all chronic hepatitis cases throughout the world. The global prevalence of chronic hepatitis C is estimated at 3%, with 150 million carriers worldwide. Five million people are infected in Europe and four million people are HCV positive in the USA,[1] where an estimated 504 new cases are contracted every day.[2] Research from 1997 estimates that the six major HCV genotypes originated at least 500 years ago and possibly as long as 2,000 years in the past.[3] The virus is transmitted through blood-to-blood contact, including unprotected sex and the sharing of needles in illicit narcotic use. A large number of cases were contracted prior to mid-1992 through tainted blood products in general hospital use. These cases are considered the most difficult to treat. HCV leads to cirrhosis, a progressive hardening of the liver similar to that in late-stage alcoholism. Although symptoms can take up to 30 years to develop, current advances have yet to counter the fatal consequences of late-stage HCV infection.

Early detection is the key to avoiding liver transplant surgery, which can prolong a patient's life for up to ten years. HCV accounts for about 1,000 liver transplants per year in the United States.

Anecdotal evidence indicates that cannabis can relieve some symptoms of hepatitis and also alleviate many adverse side effects of conventional hepatitis medications.[4] Limiting medications is imperative in managing the terminal illness, yet compassionate physicians have no compunction against approving cannabis use by HCV patients. While conventional pain medicines are frequently forbidden, patients awaiting transplant surgery are allowed to use marijuana, the safe and natural pain reliever, up to ten days prior to the operation.[5]

Related sections: *AIDS*, page 21; *Immune Responses*, page 70.

Huntington's Chorea

Huntington's Chorea is an inherited disease of the central nervous system that usually strikes adults between 30 and 50 years of age. Patients experience progressive dementia and bizarre involuntary movements including severe dystonia, slowly progressing to death. The debilitating disease has no effective medical treatment.

A stable 40% improvement in movement was documented during a two-week period by the administration of cannabidiol (CBD), a non-psychoactive cannabinoid found in natural marijuana but not in the THC pill. The 1986 study confirmed several previous scientific papers on the medical use of cannabis to control dystonic movements.[1]

Recent data from a scientist at the National Institute of Mental Health suggests that the brains of people with Huntington's Chorea lose many of their natural THC receptors early in the disease,[2] offering researchers an important clue for further investigation.

Related sections: *Cerebral Effects*, page 49; *Dystonia*, page 62; *Epilepsy*, page 62; *Multiple Sclerosis*, page 82; *Muscle Spasms*, page 83; *Neuralgia*, page 85; *Psychoactivity*, page 91; *Stroke and Head Trauma*, page 110.

Hypertension

Hypertension is the condition wherein a patient's blood pressure is deemed to be higher than normal. Hypertension is a contributing factor in many illnesses. The internal pressure exerted by the blood on the walls of the arteries and veins, called blood pressure, fluctuates with the rise and fall of physical activity. Normal blood pressure rates vary for different age and body types. High blood pressure is generally treated with weight reduction, stress management, and a reduction of salt and cholesterol in the diet.

Cannabis is known to reduce hypertension to normal levels with regular use and to maintain normal levels with continued use in some cases. Because of repeated threats by the federal government, only a few physicians have elected to recommend medical marijuana in cases of severe high blood pressure.

Related sections: *Cardiovascular Effects*, page 47; *Psychoactivity*, page 91; *Stress Reduction*, page 109.

Immune Responses

Immune Responses protect the body from disease through the development of various "defense cells," such as antibodies, macrophages, and T cells. Research on the immunological effects of cannabis use is widely contradictory. Biased researchers have often interpreted ambiguous evidence according to preconceived theories.[1] Test-tube studies finding cellular suppression of immune responses have been flawed by their use of extremely high concentrations of cannabinoids: levels impossible to attain in actual use.[2] The same flaw is found in research cited as proof that cannabinoids impair cellular metabolism.[3] Misinformed persons might consider that AIDS patients are a high-risk group for possible immune complications brought about by the use of medical marijuana, but there is no clinical or epidemiological evidence linking cannabis use to immune suppression.[4] According to cannabis researcher Leo Hollister,

> Clinically, one might assume that sustained impairment of cell-mediated immunity might lead to an increased prevalence of malignancy. No such clinical evidence has been discovered or has any direct epidemiological data incriminated marijuana use with the acquisition of human immunodeficiency virus or the clinical development of AIDS.[5]

Clinical evidence of immune suppression is somewhat contradictory. For example, N.E. Kaminsky stated in the *Journal of Neuroimmunology*, "I think there's some indication that these (cannabinoids) might be useful as relatively weak immune modulators, perhaps to be used as anti-inflammatory agents or even maybe for asthma."[6] (Asthma is thought to be an autoimmune disease.)

Research indicates that the tolerance factor found in most aspects of cannabis use probably protects the subject from potential immunological dangers. Immune suppression caused by a large overdose of cannabinoids has been shown to be reduced by repeated exposure.[7]

Several human studies of large cannabis-using populations show no difference in disease susceptibility between cannabis users and nonusers.[8] According to the United Nations World Health Organization in 1997,

> To date there has been no epidemiological evidence of increased rates of disease among chronic heavy cannabis users. Given the duration of large scale cannabis use by young adults in Western societies, the absence of any epidemics of infectious disease makes it unlikely that cannabis smoking produces major impairments in the immune system.[9]

It is possible that a small percentage of users may develop allergies to cannabinoids with repeated exposure. It is also possible that the rarely documented cases of allergic reactions to smoked cannabis have been caused by other factors such as fungi, mold, toxic insecticides, and/or herbicides. Because of the possibility of exposure to contaminant hazards, AIDS sufferers and patients with other immune deficiencies should not obtain cannabis through illegal nonmedical markets.

Related sections: *Cardiovascular Effects*, page 47; *Contaminants*, page 54; *Smoking Methods*, page 107; *Tolerance*, page 113; *Upper Respiratory Infection*, page 116.

Incarceration

Incarceration is the only well-proven health hazard associated with cannabis use. American jails are now overflowing with an estimated 1.7 million inmates, the largest per capita prison population in the world. More than 60% of those prisoners are drug offenders, many with little or no previous criminal history. Murderers and rapists frequently serve a fraction of their sentences and are free to commit more violent crimes, while nonviolent drug offenders are punished with harsh mandatory-minimum sentences. Marijuana users are subject to an average of one arrest every 49 seconds in the United States. In 1996, there were more than 650,000 Americans arrested on marijuana charges.[1] In 1997, that figure was over 700,000. In 1998, there were more arrests for marijuana possession than for all violent crimes combined.[2] The number of marijuana felons in prison in 1999 was approximately 70,000.[3] Patients suffering from severe and terminal illnesses use medicinal cannabis at the risk of intrusion into their lives and life-threatening imprisonment by social service and law enforcement agencies following the directives of "federal foolishness."[4]

While a handful of legislators, such as Congressman Barney Frank (D-MA), have sponsored several bills that would have modified existing federal statutes to exempt medical patients from prosecution, these attempts have all been defeated. In 1999, Frank introduced HR 912, which would take the matter out of the hands of the White House Office of National Drug Control Policy. Unmoved by scientific evidence and popular opinion, Drug Czar McCaffrey and policy makers at the Drug Enforcement Administration may eventually be denied their jurisdiction by Congressional Acts legalizing the use of marijuana as medicine.[5]

Until such a time as marijuana is legally defined in accordance with established medical science, federal law enforcement tactics will remain the most critical threat to the health and well-being of medical marijuana users. Studies on this issue underline the inequities of America's Drug War.[6,7] Anecdotal evidence is both poignant and compelling, such as the horror story of a wife dying of cancer while her husband is imprisoned for growing her medicine.[8] Although rescheduling marijuana for medical use was a forbidden topic in the 1999 report,[9] the Institute of Medicine's *Marijuana and Medicine* reached conclusions that clearly supported rewriting the marijuana laws enacted by Richard Nixon in 1970. Yet, regardless of the wealth of medical evidence, including the 1999 IOM recommendations, the federal government continues to enforce and escalate the war on medical marijuana,[10] forcing the closure of locally approved medical marijuana dispensaries serving tens of thousands of severely ill patients[11,12] and then prosecuting individual patients for exercising the rights granted under state law. Despite California's Compassionate Use Act and similar medical marijuana laws in other states, patients and advocates continue to suffer life-threatening incarceration by federal law enforcement agencies.[13,14]

The advent of statewide medical marijuana laws actually intensified government persecution in many conservative regions. In Los Angeles, where the new medical marijuana law was hotly denounced, the founder of a medical cannabis center, former police officer Martin Chavez, whose severe spinal injury qualifies him under California's Compassionate Use Act, was denied his legal right to a medical necessity defense and sentenced to 6 years in prison for helping sick people cope with their suffering.[15] A partner in the LA medical marijuana club, David Herrick, was sentenced to 4 years in prison for delivering small amounts of medicine to physician-approved patients.

In another graphic example of legal persecution, former gubernatorial candidate Steve Kubby and his wife Michele found picturesque Placer County in Northern California rabidly inhospitable to advocates of medical marijuana. A six-month investigation of the high-profile Libertarians resulted in the decimation of their home, even though a medical specialist confirmed that marijuana was probably responsible for Steve Kubby's continued survival of cancer. Adamantly defending their medical   qualifications under the law, the Kubbys were nonetheless charged with multiple felonies carrying a combined sentence of more than ten years in prison and more than ten thousand dollars in fines.[16]

The intent of such unjust treatment is obvious. In the words of famed linguist and social critic Noam Chomsky, "The history of the 'war on drugs,' and more specifically the well-documented history of marijuana legislation, makes it clear that the goals of the repeatedly declared 'wars' have little to do with the availability and use of harmful substances, and a lot to do with what is called 'population control.'"[17]

While medical marijuana advocates hailed the 1999 Institute of Medicine report as vindication of their cause, and while conservatives denounced it as "a thinly veiled effort to promote legalization of the drug,"[18] the million-dollar review of officially acceptable scientific studies apparently had no effect on federal policies. The US Drug Czar's office reaffirmed enforcement of laws against medical marijuana patients soon after the IOM report definitively supported rescheduling marijuana as medicine. The American Psychiatric Association newsletter, *Psychiatric News*, was sharply critical in its April 16th 1999 issue, reporting, "The White House Office of National Drug Control Policy (ONDCP) endorses the continuing arrest of medicinal marijuana users."[19] On September 13th 1999, however, the denounced federal policy was dealt a serious blow by the federal judicial system. The 9th U.S. Circuit Court of Appeals ruled that the government "has yet to identify any interest it may have in blocking the distribution of marijuana to those with medical needs. " In the landmark 3-0 ruling, the court also said that the government "has offered no evidence to rebut evidence that cannabis is the only effective treatment for a large group of seriously ill individuals."[20,21]

Insomnia

Insomnia, or chronic sleeplessness, is effectively treated with marijuana, and clinical research has verified the usefulness of marijuana in some cases. One study determined that CBD, rather than delta-9 THC, helped insomniacs sleep better. Human studies show that cannabinoid-induced sleep does not differ much from sleep induced by conventional hypnotics,[1] in contrast to one of America's favorite drugs, Valium, which, along with having a strong addictive potential, is also known to suppress stages of sleep conducive to dreaming. The Institute of Medicine recommended further study of cannabinoid sedation in its *Marijuana and Medicine* report of 1999.[2]

A small percentage of research subjects have reported unwelcome "hangover" effects following the use of cannabis as an anti-insomniac.

Related sections: *Psychoactivity*, page 91.

Intestinal Cramps

Intestinal Cramps due to many different disorders are sometimes alleviated with the use of medicinal marijuana, which relaxes tense muscles throughout the body and especially in the intestinal tract.

Related sections: *Digestive Disorders*, page 61.

Intractable Hiccups

Intractable Hiccups are a severe complication for some AIDS patients, especially in cases of esophageal candidiasis and other esophageal diseases. In 1998, the prestigious British medical journal *Lancet* published a report by physicians Gilson and Busalacchi documenting the case of an AIDS patient who underwent minor surgery that apparently triggered a severe bout of uncontrollable hiccups. The application of several different conventional treatments failed to relieve the symptoms. On the eighth day of the hiccup attack, the patient tried marijuana for the first time in his life. Amazingly, the hiccups were immediately abated. When violent hiccups returned on the following day, a second round of cannabis treatment provided permanent relief. The authors of the report concede it is unlikely that marijuana will ever be the focus of clinical trials on its effectiveness in treating intractable hiccups due to its legal prohibition.[1]

Lester Grinspoon has also noted the peculiar potential for easing hiccups with the use of cannabis in his own and in other documented cases.[2]

Marinol

Marinol is the brand name for dronabinol, the legally prescribable synthetic THC pill. In 1999, the DEA, FDA, and NIDA allowed Marinol to be re-classified from Schedule II to

Schedule III. According to the drug manufacturer, "the decision for rescheduling was greatly influenced by the findings of a study done by the Haight Ashbury Free Clinics, which concluded Marinol has a low abuse potential and that diversion is virtually non-existent."[1]

Marinol contains synthetic THC and sesame oil in a gelatin capsule. Cannabis contains natural THC and a group of interrelated compounds that are shown to have an assortment of similar therapeutic qualities. The US government approves of the use of Marinol, but rejects the medical use of marijuana. Marinol is currently a Schedule III drug, easily prescribable by physicians, but cannabis is listed in Schedule I: Simple possession is a felony punishable by imprisonment.

In 1983 the Tennessee Board of Pharmacy released a report evaluating the effects of marijuana as an antiemetic in cancer patients, reporting that, "We found both marijuana smoking and THC capsules to be effective antiemetics. We found an approximate 23 percent higher success rate among those patients smoking than among those patients administered THC capsules."[2] Similar findings are reported in other studies.[3,4] A medical journal called *Patient Care* published the following explanation of marijuana's superiority to Marinol:

> The bioavailability of dronabinol (Marinol) and marijuana vary tremendously in individuals from day to day in the same person. Even though synthetic THC is available in three strengths, it can be very difficult to define appropriate dose and determine what time of day the patient needs to take it. Some studies suggest that smoking is a more efficient delivery system for THC than dronabinol because the patient gets near immediate results and can self-titrate [control dosage].[5]

Taking Marinol is often a frustrating experience. At one time of day the medicine can seem to be completely ineffective. At another point in the patient's fluctuating rate of bioavailability, the same dose can cause intense anxiety, lightheadedness, nausea, and deep sedation. This perplexing inconsistency was the Institute of Medicine's primary criticism of Marinol in 1999.[6] The cannabis smoker's ability to determine the required dose is a critical virtue. The synthetic THC pill contains only one of 61 naturally occurring cannabinoids, some of which are known to offset the strong psychoactivity of synthetic THC. Other cannabinoids are shown to have additional and superior medical properties evidenced in other sections of this text. Although the 1999 IOM report calls for further study of all therapeutic cannabinoids, THC is the only one of those naturally occurring medicinal compounds currently available by prescription.

Another important consideration, according to the Federation of American Scientists, is the comparative price of Marinol vs. marijuana:

> Even at black-market prices, whole cannabis is substantially less expensive per bioavailable milligram of THC than is the legal synthetic, sold under the trade name Marinol.[7]

Black market sources may be more reasonable than pharmaceutical companies, but depending on outlaw drug dealers for a life-saving medication is at best a flawed proposition. Although federal drug warriors force the closure of medical marijuana clubs and co-ops, there is another alternative. High-potency cannabis rich in THC and other medicinal compounds can be a cheap renewable resource requiring only a modest investment in equipment and supplies. Comparatively, Marinol treatment usually costs thousands of dollars per month.

Meniere's Syndrome

Meniere's Syndrome is a recurrent and usually progressive group of symptoms including deafness, ringing in the ears, and a sensation of pressure in the ears. Nausea and vertigo are reported in severe cases. The cause of this debilitating illness remains unknown, and there are no effective therapies. Cannabis has been used for long-term symptomatic treatment in one case documented by physicians who authorized a patient to smoke marijuana in a Berkeley, California hospital.[1] No other medications have proved effective in relieving that patient's incapacitating symptoms.

Related sections: *Analgesia*, page 32; *Cerebral Effects*, page 49; *Neuralgia*, page 85; *Psychoactivity*, page 91.

Menstrual Cramps

Menstrual Cramps and other symptoms of severe physical discomfort often associated with menstruation have been successfully relieved by marijuana, as reported by several contemporary researchers and thousands of women. Historical medical literature abounds with specific references repeated in many diverse cultures for almost five thousand years. However, the male-dominated power structure of the current US government remains unlikely to grant serious consideration to the use of cannabis in treating this gender-specific condition.

Related sections: *Analgesia*, page 32; *Muscle Spasms*, page 83; *Obstetrics*, page 87; *Premenstrual Syndrome*, page 90.

Mental Illness

Mental Illness has been linked to the use of marijuana in a few clinical observations, particularly on populations outside of the United States. There is no clinical evidence that cannabis use directly precipitates mental illness in general, or any specific mental disorder. However, it is reasonable to assume that cannabis use might catalyze latent mental illnesses in some cases.[1] Patients suffering from severe schizophrenia, for example, should not use psychoactive medications without a physician's approval.[2] However, research from pharmacologist Daniele Piomelli in 1999 does appear to corroborate anecdotal evidence indicating that cannabinoids might help stabilize schizophrenia.

Cannabis has proven to be an effective medicine in some types of mental illness, such as major depression and bipolar disorder.[3,4]

Related sections: *Depression*, page 59; *Psychoactivity*, page 91; *Stress Reduction*, page 109.

Migraine Headaches

Migraine Headaches are severe, debilitating attacks of localized cranial pain often accompanied by distorted vision and gastrointestinal disturbance. Although little understood, migraines are thought to be caused by dilation of cranial arteries and may be associated with serotonin release from platelets in blood plasma.[1] Hotdogs and foods full of artificial preservatives are known to cause migraine attacks in some cases.[2] About 20% of the population have experienced migraines, and as many as 20% of migraine sufferers find no relief from conventional medications.

Delta-9 THC (Marinol) is clinically shown to correct serotonin release in migraine sufferers.[3] Debilitating migraine headaches are also effectively controlled by marijuana in many reported cases.[4,5] Some migraine sufferers use cannabis at the onset of a migraine attack to relieve the severe pain. Others use cannabis as a preventative measure to control migraine attacks before they occur.

Because of prohibition, only a few clinical studies of cannabis treatment for migraine have been done in recent years. However, there exists a wealth of reliable evidence in historical medical literature indicating that marijuana is effective in suppression of severe migraine headaches.[6,7,8] Cannabis medications were the most common treatment for migraine headaches until 1937 when the age-old herbal remedy was prohibited in the United States.
Related sections: *Neuralgia*, page 85; *Replacement of Medications*, page 97.

Mortality

Mortality due to cannabis use is nonexistent. Despite political assertions that marijuana is a dangerous drug, there are no cases of death directly caused by cannabis use in the entire history of human civilization. That stunning fact is further elucidated by current studies.

In 1997 the National Drug and Alcohol Research Center in Australia announced that the health of long-term marijuana users is virtually no different from that of the general population.[1] Another 1997 study from health care giant, Kaiser Permanente, published in the American Journal of Health followed 65,000 subjects during a ten-year period and concluded that "marijuana use was unassociated with non-AIDS mortality in men and was not associated with mortality in women." The report concluded that the association of marijuana with AIDS deaths probably reflects higher rates of marijuana use among the homosexual community, a group at higher risk for AIDS death irrespective of marijuana use. The comprehensive Kaiser Permanente study also found that men who smoke marijuana experience progressively diminishing mortality rates the longer they smoke.[2] In comparison, deaths due to errors in the use of prescription medications are the second most rapidly increasing cause of death after AIDS.[3]

According to The New England Journal of Medicine in 1997, "More than 65 million Americans have tried marijuana, the use of which is not associated with increased mortality."[4]

Related sections: *Replacement of Medications,* page 97; *Toxicity,* page 114.

Multiple Sclerosis

Multiple Sclerosis is a progressively degenerative nerve disease that cripples its victims and leads to death. There is no specific therapy for MS. Treatment typically consists of symptom management, commonly including steroids, tranquilizers, sedatives, barbiturates, and opiates, all of which stabilize the neurological disorder for a limited time but cause serious side effects.

Many MS patients attest that marijuana quells their uncontrollable tremors better than barbiturates and reduces the pain caused by their degenerative condition better than opiates.[1] Research confirmed that symptomatic muscle spasms were reduced by marijuana in clinical measurements of MS patients' symptoms.[2] In 1987, researchers from the UCLA School of Medicine studied 13 MS patients receiving THC in clinical trials. They concluded, "These positive findings in a treatment failure population suggest a role for THC in the treatment of spasticity in multiple sclerosis."[3]

In Britain, a majority of physicians responding to the government's call for information on medical marijuana are in favor of allowing legal access to cannabis for sufferers of multiple sclerosis.[4] The British Medical Association has asked

Parliament to speed up the processing of cannabinoid research licenses, with the highest priority given to patients with MS and other spastic disorders.[5] Geoffrey Guy was the first British researcher to be authorized to begin trials on MS patients using natural smoked marijuana. Neurologist Dennis Petro applauded these efforts, saying, "if [Dr. Guy's] studies focus on spasticity, the chances of a positive outcome are high."[6] In agreement, Roger Pertwee, President of the International Cannabinoid Research Society, remarked, "The evidence supporting the use of cannabinoids for multiple sclerosis or spinal injury is particularly promising."[7]

Multiple sclerosis sufferers often exhibit disorderly voluntary muscle coordination, called ataxia, a condition aside from pain and muscle spasms, which is also shown to be clinically improved by cannabis use in some patients.[8] Conventional antispasmodic medications used to treat the muscle spasms of MS have no anti-ataxic effect. Many of those medications have powerful side-effects that actually contribute to the debilitating symptoms of multiple sclerosis.

Related sections: *Analgesia*, page 32; *Cerebral Effects*, page 49; *Muscle Spasms*, page 83; *Neuralgia*, page 85; *Psychoactivity*, page 91; *Replacement of Medications*, page 97.

Muscle Spasms

Muscle Spasms—sudden, involuntary movements or convulsive muscular contractions—may affect many areas of the body and may be caused by numerous diseases, such as multiple sclerosis and other forms of sclerosis (hardening of tissue or nervous system), amyotrophic lateral sclerosis (Lou Gehrig's Disease), cerebral palsy, atopic neurodermitis (chronic hardening of skin), paraplegia, quadriplegia, cranial and spinal nerve injuries, and other neurological impairments such as Tourette's Syndrome and symptoms caused by stroke. In addition, asthma is in part caused by spasms of muscles coating the smaller bronchi.[1]

In several human and animal studies, natural marijuana and synthetic delta-9 THC have each been found to relieve a broad range of muscle spasms.[2,3] One 1990 double-blind trial comparing THC with codeine showed that both had an analgesic effect in comparison with a placebo, but "Only delta-9 THC showed a significant beneficial effect on spasticity."[4] Dozens of studies on human subjects have indicated that cannabis may be useful in treating various types of spastic conditions,[5,6] including cases where conventional treatments have failed.[7]

Some patients find that cannabis is invaluable in alleviating the chronic debilitation of their uncontrollable muscle tremors.[8] Patients suffering from severe spastic conditions have reported that cannabis actually keeps them alive.[9] According to pharmacologist Daniele Piomelli, there is strong clinical evidence that the anandamide-boosting properties of THC might help alleviate symptoms of Tourette's Syndrome.[10] Even the conservative American Medical Association has agreed: "Anecdotal, survey, and clinical data support the view that smoked marijuana and oral THC provide symptomatic relief in some patients with spasticity associated with multiple sclerosis or trauma."[11]

Unlike natural cannabis, powerful barbiturates and muscle relaxers currently in use for treatment of severe muscle spasms are known to have serious and life-threatening side effects.

Related sections: *Multiple Sclerosis*, page 82; *Neuralgia*, page 85; *Replacement of Medications*, page 97.

Neuralgia

Neuralgia is a broad term for nerve injuries characterized by sharp pain or other neural symptoms such as convulsive tics and tic douloureux. Spinal injury is one common cause of severe and crippling neuralgia.[1] Cranial nerve damage can also create crippling neuralgic symptoms.[2] Most forms of neuralgia are usually found to be at least partially relieved by the use of marijuana. General analgesic properties of cannabis have been noted for millennia, but modern science has determined that the cannabinoids actually govern the body's neurological pain control mechanisms.[3,4,5]

Cannabis has been cited by many sufferers to be a superior medication in severe neuralgic conditions, compared to commonly prescribed drugs such as sedatives, tranquilizers, opiates, and painkillers, all of which suppress neurological functions. Using narcotics to treat pain associated with nerve injury is ineffective and frequently contributes to neuralgic symptoms.

Related sections: *Addiction*, page 29; *Analgesia*, page 32; *Cerebral Effects*, page 49; *Muscle Spasms*, page 83; *Neurodermitis*, page 86; *Psychoactivity*, page 91; *Replacement of Medications*, page 97.

Neurodermitis

Neurodermitis (atopic) is a severe skin disease that is both debilitating and potentially life threatening. There is no cure for the disease. Prescribed therapies are aimed at relieving the irritation of progressively hardening skin tissue. Atopic neurodermitis is one of the conditions relieved by cannabis medications in testimony put before DEA Administrative Law Judge Francis Young. In 1988, after months of testimony, Young handed down an historic ruling allowing prescriptive access to marijuana. Young's ruling was summarily denied by federal Drug Enforcement Administration authorities.[1]

Related sections: *Neuralgia*, page 85.

Nutrition

Nutrition is a subject apart from medical research on the therapeutic effects of cannabis compounds. However, as some patients ingest whole marijuana in brownies or other foods, it bears noting that cannabis seeds are highly nutritious. Essential fatty acids, B vitamins, and complete proteins found in hemp seeds have served as one of mankind's oldest renewable food sources.[1,2,3,4,5] While drug-testing agencies lobby to ban all hemp products, the US Food and Drug Administration has no objection to nonnutritive food additives such as monosodium glutamate and the recently developed Olestra, which do have known health hazards.[6]

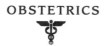
Obstetrics

Obstetrics, the care of women in childbirth, includes one of the oldest and most well-known medical applications of cannabis. Pregnancy is frequently marked by nausea and vomiting, commonly called "morning sickness." Marijuana is famous for its antinausea and appetite stimulating properties. Increased food consumption is generally thought to provide greater health for both mother and fetus through all stages of pregnancy. Marijuana is also known to reduce physical discomfort both as an anti-inflammatory agent and as an analgesic, thereby also decreasing the stress characteristic of pregnancy. And marijuana is historically reported to ease the pain of childbirth by relaxing uterine contractions. Prior to 1970, when America became subject to a sharp increase of antimarijuana propaganda, the effects of cannabis during labor were openly discussed in the Journal of the *American Medical Association*:

> The sensation of pain is distinctly lessened or entirely absent and the sense of touch is less acute than normally. Hence a woman in labor may have a more or less painless labor. If a sufficient amount of the drug is taken, the patient may fall into a tranquil sleep from which she will awaken refreshed. As far as is known, a baby born of a mother intoxicated with cannabis will not be abnormal in any way.[1]

In analyzing the many conflicting studies on birth weight, length of term, and teratogenicity (birth defects), the current weight of evidence suggests that cannabis does not harm the human fetus.[2] Most health experts do, however, urge caution in the use of cannabis during pregnancy. Australian health authorities have remarked that, " . . . given the uncertainty about the validity of self-reported cannabis use in many of the null studies [showing no evidence of birth defects], it would be unwise to exonerate cannabis as a cause of birth defects until larger, better controlled studies have been conducted."[3] A similar caution is expressed by cannabis researcher Leo Hollister:

> While no definite clinical association has yet been made between cannabis use during pregnancy and fetal abnormalities, such events are likely to be rare and could be easily missed. The belated recognition of the harmful effects on the fetus of smoking tobacco and drinking alcoholic beverages indicates that some caution with cannabis is wise.[4]

In contrast to the caution and reservations expressed by research scientists, well-controlled field studies conclude that cannabis use is not harmful to mother or developing fetus. A study published by the American Academy of Pediatrics in 1994 sought to clarify previous research on prenatal use of cannabis that was considered inconclusive and conflicting.[5] A highly controlled study titled *Prenatal Marijuana Exposure and Neonatal Outcomes in Jamaica: an Ethnographic Study* conclusively determined that the offspring of prenatal marijuana users had significantly higher test scores on habituation to auditory and tactile stimulation; their degree of alertness was higher; their capacity for consolability was higher; and they had fewer startles and tremors during the first week following birth. At thirty days after birth, the offspring of prenatal marijuana users had a higher quality of alertness; their voluntary and involuntary reflex systems were more robust; they were less irritable; and they were more adept at organization than the offspring of nonusing mothers with similar cultural and economic backgrounds.[6,7]

A similar finding is noted in the 1997 birth of a healthy child to a cannabis-using mother in the United States. Keeping careful records of daily cannabis consumption during term, the mother discovered that the moderate use of marijuana to relieve pain and physical stress had great benefits to herself and no adverse effects on the newborn. Increased cannabis use by the mother following childbirth was also found to have no adverse effects. (Clinical evidence shows that metabolized cannabinoids enter the milk of breastfeeding mothers.) Medical examination of the infant showed all areas of development well within normal ranges one year following delivery.[8]

Don Wirtshafter, owner of The Ohio Hempery, the largest hemp trading company in America, provides a well-documented report on the use of cannabis in birthing. The mother, Christine Wirtshafter, used nutritional treatments that included hemp seeds and hemp seed oil to provide protein, vitamins, minerals, and essential fatty acids to the growing fetus. Hempseed oil was applied for perineal massage. A difficult birth lasting approximately 36 hours was greatly relieved with ingestion of medicinal cannabis. The child, named Sativa, was born in 1994. Mother and child continue in good health.[9]

Warning: although cannabis has been used as a medical treatment in obstetrics for thousands of years in most parts of the world, cannabis prohibition in the United States can endanger the health of mothers and infants testing positive for cannabinoids in conservative medical practices. In all cases, the physician in charge should be aware of adjunctive medications prior to any complications arising from legal issues. Mothers have been known to lose custody of their children for testing positive for cannabinoids.[10] In another case, a traditional midwife practice in Santa Cruz was shut down for possession of marijuana.[11]

Related sections: *Analgesia*, page 32; *Arthritis*, page 40; *Chromosome Interference*, page 53; *Digestive Disorders*, page 61; *Fertility*, page 63; *Marinol*, page 76; *Muscle Spasms*, page 83; *Premenstrual Syndrome*, page 90; *Sexual Activity*, page 107.

Paranoia Attacks

Paranoia Attacks have been reported clinically and by a small percentage of casual users. A person predisposed to paranoid thinking may be adversely antagonized by the psychoactive properties of cannabis, however, the legal status of the drug is probably the most pervasive factor in development of marijuana-induced paranoia. With the exception of a realistic concern for legal issues, all psychological effects of cannabis are limited to a maximum of several hours following consumption.

Related sections: *Anxiety Attacks*, page 39; *Psychoactivity*, page 91.

Premenstrual Syndrome

Premenstrual Syndrome, or PMS, refers to the irritability, emotional tension, anxiety, depression, headaches, and physical discomfort that often occur several days before the onset of menstruation. Anecdotal evidence suggests that cannabis use may reduce pain in severe cases of PMS.

Related sections: *Menstrual Cramps*, page 79; *Muscle Spasms*, page 83; *Obstetrics*, page 87; *Stress Reduction*, page 109.

Psychoactivity

Psychoactivity refers to the mental effects of some medications. Subjective experiences of being "high" on marijuana may seem as varied as the persons who report them, yet there are some commonalities. Typically, the psychoactivity of cannabis is unobtrusive; first-time users frequently fail to notice any difference in their perceptions. With repeated use the psychoactive effects are learned.

There have been many literary descriptions of cannabis intoxication, both graphic and poetic.[1] A heightened sense of mental flow is almost universal. Psychoactivity seems to turn up the "volume" or "brightness" of the mind's internal dialogue. Sensory perceptions are heightened as the nervous system becomes subtly charged with an added intensity. Intuitive understanding becomes more easily accessible. Unbridled hilarity and a pronounced sense of innate profundity may infuse the mind with compelling expressions.

The psychotropic effects of cannabis vary widely with differences in dosage, potency, method of ingestion, individual differences in metabolism, and relative experience of the user. For one who is familiar with the effects, a few puffs of smoke can pleasantly blend perception and experience in a clear and cohesive associative understanding that may not be obvious to a nonuser. On the other hand, a very large dose orally ingested by an inexperienced subject can result in a temporary panic or induce mental confusion, usually followed by deep sedation. THC intoxication can sometimes induce mild visual imagery to swirl and dance behind closed eyes. Although sensations can be intensified to an uncomfortable level by psychoactive excess, true hallucinations or radically altered perceptions are extremely rare and easily averted.

The mild mental stimulation of a normal dose of cannabis can be useful in increasing the attention span and mental concentration. That same mental stimulation can cause an undisciplined mind to wander aimlessly. One might become more absorbed with a project or task using normal doses of cannabis. A much larger dose might induce the same individual to abandon the task and drift in contemplation. While contemplation may be intuitively invaluable under some conditions, associative musings can certainly prove detrimental to students at test time.

Marijuana can exaggerate and intensify preexisting moods. A tired person might feel sleepy, but a more rested person might feel mentally stimulated by the same dose of marijuana. External variables also contribute to the subjective effects. Timothy Leary stressed the value of "set and setting" in the psychology of psychoactive drug experiences. In group use, marijuana tends to increase a person's susceptibility to the moods of other people, enhancing social harmony.[2]

Physiological symptoms such as an increased heart rate may correlate with the mental and sensory excitement often experienced immediately following administration. This mild increase in heart rate is generally self-correcting within 20 to 40 minutes, and mental excitement steadily diminishes accordingly.

Trace elements of cannabinoids are absorbed by and stored in the fatty tissues of the body. Although detectable by various drug-testing methods for several weeks following ingestion, these metabolized trace elements are definitely not psychoactive.[3] Although some occasional users may report a mild "hangover" the following day, all notable effects of cannabis wear off within a few hours following administration.[4]

Deeper understandings and a deeper appreciation of art and music are frequently ascribed to cannabis use. Artistic expression is also said to be heightened, which can be interpreted as an increase in associative rather than linear thought patterns. Some researchers have occasionally noted mild episodes of psychoactive *déjà vu*. The link between cannabis and associative thinking is also indicated by the discovery of cannabinoid receptor sites located in the right frontal lobe of the brain, which governs memory and emotion.[5]

Chronic users, such as patients who consume one or more grams per day over a period of many months or years, universally report that the psychoactive effects of cannabis diminish in proportion to continued use. With continued exposure, the mental stimulation experienced by occasional users is gradually transformed to an overall sensation that may be expressed as a glow of warmth or comfort insulating the patient from a general or specific pain or discomfort. When cannabis is used as an analgesic, patients frequently report that their pain fades away or becomes more distant. These subtle effects contrast greatly with the complete sensory suppression characteristic of opiate narcotic painkillers.

While law enforcement officials incorrectly classify marijuana as a hallucinogenic drug, established medical literature accurately classifies marijuana as a euphoriant.[6] Many cannabis users feel a heightened sense of self-awareness contributing to a greater feeling of well-being—the literal definition of euphoria.

Related sections: *Analgesia*, page 32; *Anxiety Attacks*, page 39; *Cerebral Effects*, page 49; *Stress Reduction*, page 109; *Tolerance*, page 113.

Psychomotor Skills

Psychomotor Skills of persons under the influence of cannabis, such as the ability to operate an automobile, have been studied more thoroughly than most of the potential medical benefits covered in this book. Despite efforts to blame cannabis for a large number of highway fatalities and other auto accidents, a thorough analysis of available data supports the contention that psychomotor skills are not significantly impaired by typical doses of marijuana.

In 1990, the US National Transportation Safety Board (NTSB) reported that 12.8% of those involved in fatal truck accidents showed signs of cannabis use in postmortem examination. However, that statistic is an unreliable indicator of the effects of cannabis on driving performance because other drugs, particularly alcohol, were present in a majority of those cases. A much larger NTSB study published in 1988 found that those drivers using only cannabis accounted for 2.2% of fatal accidents. That report concluded, "THC plays a relatively minor role in fatal traffic accidents as compared with alcohol."[1]

In 1992, a study was released by the National Highway Transportation Safety Administration (NHTSA) indicating that alcohol is by far the leading cause of drug-related traffic accidents, while marijuana poses a negligible danger, except when combined with alcohol. In an analysis of blood samples from 1,882 drivers killed in vehicular accidents in seven states, alcohol was found in over 51%. Marijuana was a distant second to alcohol at just 6.7%. Because two-thirds of those deceased marijuana users were also under the influence of alcohol at the time of death, the actual number of drivers who tested positive for cannabis was 2.2%, the exact number determined by the NTSB in 1988. The US government's 1992 NHTSA research, considered the most comprehensive study of cannabis use among driving fatalities, was suppressed for almost two years because it contradicted America's "just say no" propaganda.[2] The irrationality of marijuana prohibition becomes plain upon realization that drunk drivers are more than seven and one-half times more likely to die in auto accidents than are marijuana users who don't drink and drive. Then again, even that statistic is misleading because testing positive for marijuana use does not prove that the subject was "high" at the moment of impact. While alcohol leaves the body quickly over the course of a few hours, cannabinoids are stored in fat cells of the body and may be detected up to five weeks following consumption. Cannabis users continue to test positive long past the time of intoxication. There is no evidence that any of those drivers who died at the wheel with cannabinoids in their system were actually under the influence of marijuana at the time of death. Considering that drinking and driving is the leading cause of death in 18- to 24-year-old Americans, the contrast between "acceptable limits" of alcohol inebriation and "zero tolerance" of marijuana use is sheer hypocrisy.

In 1996, the National Highway Transportation Safety Administration published results of the University of Lindburg study in the Netherlands under the title Marijuana and Actual Driving Performance.[3] In the introduction of that paper, a review of previously published data on traffic accidents involving cannabis use was again declared inconclusive due to the prevalence of other substances; 60-80% of drivers who were found positive for cannabis also tested positive for alcohol. As these statistics are an unreliable indicator of the affect of cannabis intoxication on motor skills, Hindrik Robbe and his team of researchers conducted exhaustive testing of actual performance of drivers while they were under the influence of cannabis. Drivers were tested both on highways and in urban traffic. Driving performance was rated by licensed driving instructors. The US National Institute on Drug Abuse supplied marijuana cigarettes and nonintoxicating placebo "joints." Comprehensive urine analysis was conducted to determine actual levels of THC intoxication in two dozen 21- to 40-year-old test subjects. The well-controlled scientific study concluded,

> This program of research has shown that marijuana produces only a moderate degree of driving impairment which is related to the consumed THC dose. The impairment manifests itself mainly in the ability to maintain a steady lateral position on the road, but its magnitude is not exceptional in comparison with changes produced by many medicinal drugs and alcohol. Drivers under the influence of marijuana retain insight into their performance and will compensate when they can (e.g., by increasing distance between vehicles or increasing effort). As a consequence, THC's adverse effects on driving performance appeared relatively small in the tests employed in this program.[4]

Most studies of actual driving ability do show that psychomotor skills are mildly impaired at high doses of delta-9 THC, especially when it is taken by inexperienced subjects. Subjects familiar with the effects of cannabis use generally show less impairment, and in some cases, experienced marijuana users have shown a documented increase in psychomotor skills while under the influence of THC.[5] All major research on the subject indicates that the effects of cannabis and synthetic delta-9 THC have minimal effects on psychomotor skills as compared to the effects of alcohol, barbiturates, opiate compounds, and some over-the-counter medications.

The US National Traffic Highway Safety Administration has determined that the only major statistical outcome associated with marijuana use in driving is a mild degree of speed reduction, a finding noted by Hindrik Robbe in the Netherlands. Speed reduction is a classic symptom of cannabis intoxication, which was also reported in the United Nations World Health Organization report on the probable health effects of cannabis. In the suppressed UN report of 1997, the World Health Organization concluded that "No controlled epidemiological studies have established that cannabis users are at increased risk of motor vehicle accidents."[6]

Also in 1997, a psychiatrist named Lehman, with over 60 years of medical practice under his belt, testified before a Canadian court in the case of Ontario hemp store owner Chris Clay. In that doctor's opinion, "A driver talking on a cellular phone is more of a menace on the road than one who has just smoked a marijuana joint."[7]

Related sections: *Cerebral Effects*, page 49; *Psychoactivity*, page 91.

Replacement of Medications

Replacement of Medications legally prescribed by physicians is a common trend among the majority of medical marijuana users. Recent studies indicate that the replacement of legal medications with the remarkably safe alternative of medicinal cannabis may greatly increase a patient's longevity. According to an overview of research published in the *Journal of the American Medical Association* in 1998, bad reactions to prescription and over-the-counter medications kill more than 100,000 Americans per year and seriously injure an additional 2.1 million. The article's author, Dr. Bruce Pomeranz, wrote that these deaths and other permanent injuries are not caused by medical errors or drug abuse. Blame was laid on the drugs themselves; virtually all medications can have serious side effects and some are fatal even in recommended doses. Pomeranz and colleagues estimated that 7% of all hospital admissions in the United States are due to bad reactions to legal medications. Low estimates rank adverse reactions to legal medications as the sixth leading cause of death in the United States.[1] Of great concern to patients is the fact that the instances of prescription-related deaths more than doubled in American patients during the period 1983 to 1993.[2]

Aside from death and permanent injury, most legal prescription medications have unwanted side effects that can radically undermine a patient's quality of life. Although a small percentage of patients in clinical trials and research studies report that the psychoactive side effects of THC are not always well tolerated, these side effects usually diminish with repeated use. (See Tolerance.) One of eighty-five legally prescribable psychoactive drugs in the standard pharmacopoeia,[3] delta-9 THC (Marinol) is often said to be too powerful in present forms.[4] However, the health risks of THC intoxication, whether the substance is ingested in pill form or smoked as whole marijuana, are minimal compared to the side effects of many pharmaceutical medications.

Compazine, a drug used to control severe nausea, psychotic disorders, and nonpsychotic anxiety, is known to produce irreversible Tardive Dyskinesia—a loss of control over voluntary muscles—and symptoms similar to those of Parkinson's Disease.[5] In turn, Levodopa, the drug most commonly used to treat Parkinson's Disease, is recently shown to produce visual and auditory hallucinations.[6] Popular medicines such as the entire range of widely prescribed Non-Steroid Anti-Inflammatory Drugs, (NSAIDs) are the cause of over 7,600 deaths and 70,000 hospitalizations per year.[7] A common migraine medication, Cafergot, is a vasodilator that can cause gangrene. A newer migraine medication, Imitrex, causes severe chest pains. Thorazine is a standard tranquilizer used to treat psychotic disorders, nausea and vomiting, restlessness, porphyria (sometimes caused by the use of sulfonamides, barbiturates, or other drugs), tetanus, manic-depressive illness, intractable hiccups, severe behavior problems, and migraine headaches. Thorazine is another drug known to cause Tardive Dyskinesia, a syndrome of potentially irreversible loss of muscle control. Thorazine also causes Neuroplectic Malignant Syndrome, with symptoms including high fever, muscle stiffness, altered mental status, irregular pulse, extreme heart rate, and death.[8] A potent new painkiller, Duract, is known to produce potentially fatal liver damage.[9] Rezulin, a new pill for treating diabetes, is also know to cause fatal liver damage. Rezulin was used by more than one million patients, even after FDA physicians admitted that "the agency initially overlooked compelling evidence of its danger to the liver."[10] The popular impotence pill, Viagra, the largest-selling drug in US history, caused at least six deaths in the first month of FDA-approved use.[11] As of this writing, hundreds of people have died from using the new sex drug. Viagra is also known to cause retinal dysfunction, and some users have reported blue-tinted vision and vivid hallucinations.[12] These examples represent thousands of adverse reactions to legal medications, many of which are listed in the Physician's Desk Reference of Pharmaceutical Products as well as in after-market health warnings issued by drug manufacturers.

Even common over-the-counter medicines have associated dangers: aspirin is known to cause stomach bleeding and about 1,000 American deaths per year.[13] Acetaminophen, (Tylenol) a common replacement for aspirin, is linked to liver and kidney failure with continued use.[14] Five times the recommended dose of Tylenol would "unequivocally produce a life-threatening injury in anybody," according to Eugene Schiff, director of the Center for Liver Diseases at the University of Miami School of Medicine. William Lee, professor of Internal Medicine at the University of Texas also warns patients about the dangers of Tylenol, declaring that, "no over-the-counter drug has a narrower range between therapy and toxicity than acetaminophen." The number of deaths attributable to Tylenol is higher than the number of deaths due to cocaine overdose.[15]

In general, drugs that suppress the nervous system tend to cause psychological depression and severely inhibit mental clarity. Addictive drugs such as benzodiazepines, opiates, and opiate derivatives can create far-reaching psychological consequences, often leading to a distinct shift in personal values centered around consumption of the substance. While these side effects are currently recognized, many more unwelcome effects may become obvious over the course of continued use. Every patient should be aware that 90% of the medications in use today have been introduced into the human body only within the last 30 years; there is absolutely no data available on long-term use.[16] At the end of the twentieth century, nearly all of the drugs prescribed by physicians have been in use for less than half of an average human life. In comparison, over a documented history of 5,000 years, cannabis has been shown to be one of the safest and most widely used therapeutic agents known to mankind. A complete review of marijuana studies during the drug war years prompted Dr. Lester Grinspoon to conclude, "The years of effort devoted to showing marijuana is exceedingly dangerous have proved the opposite."[17]

Why has the US government spent vast fortunes in a vain attempt to identify the destructive effects of this innocuous herb? With the use of cannabis as a replacement for dangerous medications, pharmaceutical companies are losing huge profits. In 1998, more than 2.8 billion prescriptions were filled—more than eleven for every man, woman, and child in the United States. Economic incentives fuel the federal ban on medical marijuana, a renewable source of unpatentable medicines. Medications commonly replaced by cannabis include antiemetics, anticonvulsants, antidepressants, barbiturates, hypnotics, insulin,[18] muscle relaxers, nonsteroid anti-inflammatory drugs, steroid drugs, tranquilizers, sedatives, opiate and nonopiate painkillers, and many other medications known to have serious health risks.

Note: The physician in charge should be informed of all medication adjustments, even in light of federal and state anti-marijuana laws.

Related sections: *Addiction*, page 29; *Cancer*, page 42; *Psychoactivity*, page 91; *Toxicity*, page 114.

Respiratory Diseases

Respiratory Diseases are often cited as the major health threat of smoked marijuana. Some studies have attempted to prove that marijuana smoke contains carcinogenic materials and leads to lung damage as does tobacco smoke.[1] Such research often fails to provide adequate controls, as in a 1972 study of US servicemen who smoked hashish and tobacco. A review of the published data reveals that not a single case of lung cancer has ever been attributed to marijuana smoke.[2]

Comparing tobacco smoking to marijuana smoking only reveals that marijuana smoke is relatively harmless. As has been noted by the National Academy of Sciences, 50 to 60 million American tobacco smokers produce about 150,000 cases of lung cancer per year. If marijuana smoking were equally dangerous, then the estimated 10 to 15 million current marijuana smokers in America should produce in the range of 30 to 40 thousand lung cancer cases, but again, not even one such case has ever been reported.[3]

The argument that cannabis smoke may be as hazardous as tobacco smoke is weakened by the disparity in quantity of material smoked and also by the lack of epidemiological evidence. A patient suffering from a chronic condition might inhale in the range of three grams of medicinal marijuana per day.[4,5] Comparatively, the typical tobacco addict who smokes twenty or more cigarettes per day consumes about four to five times that amount of plant material. The actual amount of smoke produced is in the range of seven times greater for cigarette smokers than for heavy marijuana smokers.[6] While it usually takes a chronic tobacco addict twenty years to develop lung cancer, it would take a marijuana smoker at least eighty years of constant chronic use to develop lung cancer, if cannabis smoke were as dangerous as tobacco.[7]

Any comparisons between cannabis and tobacco are seriously flawed in that the respiratory effects of the two materials are distinctly different. Cannabis smoke is known to be a bronchial dilator that helps clear the larger central airways of the lung, while tobacco smoke is known to penetrate the lung's smaller peripheral air passages, causing blockages and leading to emphysema.[8] Tashkin, a leading pulmonary expert with UCLA, has conducted what UCSF researcher Abrams called "elegant" research indicating that cannabinoids actually protect human lungs from diseased conditions such as emphysema.[9,10] In 1994 Donald Tashkin, federally sponsored pulmonologist and professor of medicine at UCLA, lectured on his study of habitual marijuana smokers. He concluded that marijuana smokers do not face the same degree of lung injury as tobacco addicts. Tashkin cited two main reasons. First, in the population he studied, tobacco smokers inhaled an average of 25 cigarettes per day, compared to heavy marijuana users who smoked an average of 3 or 4 marijuana "joints" per day—a sevenfold difference in the amount of smoke inhaled. Second, there is a qualitative difference between tobacco and marijuana smoke. Extensive testing determined that marijuana smoke does not precipitate the same destructive changes to lung tissue as does tobacco smoke. Marijuana and tobacco smoke may both contain toxic compounds; however, unlike cannabis, tobacco smoke causes inflammation of the lung's absorbent macrophages. This evidence led Dr. Tashkin to theorize that marijuana smoke may actually release compounds known to suppress inflammation of the lung's macrophages, thereby blocking the absorption of toxic substances.[11]

Whereas marijuana in medical use is often criticized because it is known to contain about 421 interrelated compounds, tobacco cigarettes contain more than 4,000 ingredients.[12] More than a half million Americans per year die from tobacco-related illnesses, but not one death has ever been attributed to smoking cannabis. In 1990, the 20th edition of the California Research Advisory Panel annual report declared that "An objective consideration of marijuana shows that it is responsible for less damage to society and the individual than are alcohol and cigarettes."[13] In 1997, the United Nations World Health Organization published an identical declaration. Unfortunately, public release of that comprehensive report was suppressed in the United States.[14]

A survey by the Kaiser Permanente Center found that marijuana-only smokers have a 19% higher rate of respiratory complaints than nonsmokers.[15] An early paper by Donald Tashkin reported evidence of minor lung damage caused by frequent marijuana smoking.[16] In the US government's 1999 review of scientific literature, the Institute of Medicine considered these and similar published reports. In assessing this aspect of medical marijuana, the IOM Executive Summary notes that, "Numerous studies suggest that marijuana smoke is an important risk factor in the development of respiratory disease."[17] Yet the IOM report apparently failed to consider a number of recent studies that clearly contradict the assertion that marijuana smoke is a risk factor for respiratory disease. Harvard Medical Professor Lester Grinspoon, M.D., states that the IOM report, "greatly exaggerated" the risks of smoking marijuana.[18] Many other physicians and medical researchers have reported that even long-term inhalation of marijuana smoke does not cause any type of lung disease.

A 1992 paper studied the effects of cannabis on ventilatory drive and metabolic rate in 11 young, healthy marijuana-only smoking men. There was no evidence of hypercapnia (increased carbon dioxide in the blood) or hypoxia (lowered oxygen in the blood). To quote the study, "We conclude that smoking marijuana (13 to 27 mg THC) has no acute effect on central or peripheral ventilatory drive or metabolic rate in habitual marijuana smokers."[19] Also in 1992, the National Academy of Science reported a similar finding. "Other than brochiodilation, it has proven difficult to demonstrate any effects of acute cannabis smoking on breathing as measured by conventional pulmonary [respiratory] testing."[20]

In 1997, a UCLA team headed by Tashkin concluded an extensive study of 394 participants. Comprehensive analysis found that habitual long-term marijuana smokers do not experience a greater decline in lung function than nonsmokers. Researchers remarked, "Neither the continuing nor the intermittent marijuana smokers exhibited any significantly different rates of decline in [lung function]. No differences were noted between even quite heavy marijuana smoking and nonsmoking of marijuana." In contrast, the tobacco-only smokers in the study experienced a rapid decline in lung function during the 8 years of pulmonary examination. The study also found no connection between marijuana and tobacco in those who smoked both. The evidence from this exhaustive, real-world study indicates that the pulmonary health of marijuana smokers is no different from that of the general population.[21]

A 1995 editorial in The Lancet, the premiere medical journal in Britain, opened with this definitive assessment: "The smoking of cannabis, even long term, is not harmful to health."[22] The respected UK medical authority published a more thorough analysis of marijuana's harmful effects in 1998. Editors of The Lancet concluded that "moderate indulgence in cannabis has little ill effect."[23] These findings are similar to those presented by the United Nations World Health Organization in 1997 in the report that was officially suppressed in the United States.[24]

US Drug Czars refuse to recognize accepted medical research and instead cite questionable government studies showing that cannabis smoke contains carcinogens and therefore must cause lung cancer.[25] Their assertions make effective media "sound bytes," but lose their power upon exposure to the facts. It is well known that marijuana available for study from the National Institute on Drug Abuse (NIDA) is not satisfactory for medical use. Researchers and patients receiving cannabis grown by the federal government have learned to remove a large percentage of unsmokable plant materials— seeds, stems, and unknown substances—prior to smoking or eating.[26,27] It is doubtful that researchers cleaned the inferior government-grown marijuana before burning it to identify smoke by-products in antimarijuana studies funded by the National Institute on Drug Abuse. Even granting consideration to the questionable data touted by Drug Czars, the 1999 Institute of Medicine report was cautious to qualify its judgement on the potential risk for lung damage. Discrediting alarmist propaganda, the IOM report concluded, ". . . proof that habitual marijuana smoking does or does not cause cancer awaits the results of well-designed studies."[28]

Unfortunately, federal censorship prevented the IOM investigators from assessing the implications of the suppressed National Toxicology Program study referred to in the *Cancer* section of this book.[29] That study supports the claims of cancer survivors who attribute some aspect of their remission to continued use of medical marijuana.

In reviewing pulmonary hazards associated with marijuana smoke, the mode of administration is a critical factor that is frequently ignored. It is important to note the recent development of vaporizer technology. Because the ignition temperature of THC is much lower than that required to ignite plant material, modern vaporizers offer a potentially safer method of inhaled administration. However, this health-conscious technology is severely restricted by "drug paraphernalia" ordinances prohibiting sale and promotion of illegal merchandise. As with prohibition of needle-exchange programs for IV drug users, the illegal status of the drug only contributes to its potential for harm.

Another significant factor in assessing pulmonary hazards is the strength of the marijuana. The 1987 edition of the Merck manual of pharmaceutical drugs stated that marijuana used in the United States does in fact have higher THC content than in former years. Critics have incorporated this observation into warnings, but the fact is that the health risks of smoking cannabis are lower with the higher-potency marijuana available today than they were back when people were smoking a relatively inferior grade. Low-potency marijuana requires much greater consumption and certainly increases any potential respiratory health risks. Marijuana leaf, or "shake," is usually of minimal potency and burns hotter than the dense flowering tops, frequently causing coughing fits upon deep inhalation.

Marijuana used for clinical research in assessing the risk of associated lung damage is notoriously inferior to cannabis obtained through medical marijuana groups or the black market. Marijuana supplied by the National Institute on Drug Abuse is only about 25% as potent as average grades of medical cannabis used, for example, in San Francisco Bay Area medical cannabis clubs. The Institute of Medicine report of 1999 cites the risk of smoking as the one notable health hazard of cannabis consumption, yet patients receiving cannabis grown by the government through research studies and through the Compassionate Use Investigational New Drugs Program face 4 to 5 times greater exposure to potential smoke hazards than do the many thousands of patients who procure their medicine through illegal cannabis dispensaries.[30]

Patients concerned with potential risks of cannabis smoke may completely circumvent the respiratory system by utilizing various methods of oral ingestion.

Related sections: *Cancer*, page 42; *Immune Responses*, page 70; *Smoking Methods*, page 107; *Upper Respiratory Infection*, page 116.

Sexual Activity

Sexual Activity is usually enhanced by cannabis. Historical records document the aphrodisiac properties of marijuana in many different cultures. A study by sex researchers Masters and Johnson found that cannabis enhanced sex for most users. Of 1,000 cannabis users surveyed, 83% of men and 81% of woman reported that cannabis enhanced their sexual experiences.[1]

Related sections: *Fertility*, page 63; *Psychoactivity*, page 91.

Smoking Methods

Smoking Methods and materials vary widely among cannabis users. Gauging the effects of marijuana smoke on the lungs and respiratory system is extremely difficult due to the wide variety of smoking techniques. The many variables apparent in evaluating the respiratory risks of smoking cannabis include not only the method of inhalation but also the potency and purity of the product consumed.

Smoking properly cultivated, high-potency cannabis using a dual-action hot/cold water pipe may lessen tar intake without reducing delivery of medicinal compounds, according to Lester Grinspoon, M.D. Conventional water pipes, however, do little to lower the ratio of tar to THC. The hand-rolled cigarette (joint), presents a much lesser health risk than do to all types of conventional pipes. Marijuana cigarettes burn at lower temperatures than most pipes, reducing the potential for heat damage to respiratory tissues. With the advent of hemp rolling papers, even the questionable residue of wood paper may be avoided. In the future, developments in vaporizer technology offer a potentially risk-free method of inhalation by vaporizing medicinal cannabinoids without burning the plant material.[1] Unfortunately, legal complications and enforced ignorance stymie this harm-reduction technology. Dr. Grinspoon submitted information to the Institute of Medicine on prototype vaporizers prior to its *Marijuana and Medicine* report, yet, in the words of Tod Mikuriya, M.D., the federal government's highest medical authority "pointedly chose to omit" any reference to the smokeless marijuana vaporizers.[2]

Cannabis prohibition severely cripples both scientific research and public information on risk-free smoking methods. Additionally, legislation outlawing "drug paraphernalia" reduces public access to safer smoking techniques. To complicate the matter even further, popular media portrayals commonly support the misconception that marijuana smokers should inhale deeply and hold the smoke in the lungs for as long as possible to gain the greatest effect. While novice smokers might mistake the symptoms of hyperventilation for the subtle psychoactive qualities of THC, experienced cannabis users eventually discover that all smoking methods are more advantageous when performed with less vigor.

Cannabinoids are fat-soluble and readily absorbed by the respiratory system, entering the bloodstream almost immediately upon contact. In fact, cannabinoids are so easily assimilated that second-hand smoke can cause one to test positive in a urinary drug screening after just 20 minutes of passive exposure.[3,4,5] Tars and other smoke by-products, on the other hand, are not fat-soluble and require comparatively prolonged saturation to penetrate soft lung tissue. Therefore, inhaling deeply and holding the smoke in the lungs for more than a few seconds is not only useless, it also causes greater exposure to toxic substances. To achieve the greatest medical benefits of inhaled cannabis smoke, then, the optimum method is a few seconds of moderate inhalation.

Note: an advisable regimen for patients concerned about potential health risks associated with smoking cannabis includes the daily intake of a multiple B-complex vitamin supplement and a basic antioxidant formula including one mixed carotene supplement, 400-800 IU of natural vitamin E, 200 micrograms of selenium, and 1,000 to 2,000 mg of vitamin C taken two to three times per day.[6]

Any potentially deleterious effects of cannabis smoke may be completely avoided through various methods of oral ingestion.

Related sections: *Cancer*, page 42; *Contaminants*, page 54; *Immune Responses*, page 70; *Respiratory Disease*, page 101; *Toxicity*, page 114; *Upper Respiratory Infection*, page 116.

Stress Reduction

Stress Reduction is a nearly universal benefit of cannabis use. Psychiatrist Tod Mikuriya, M.D., notes, "Continued use [of marijuana] exhibits a much more controlled pattern of mood management through a mild stimulation with low repeated inhaled doses."[1] Scientific research supports the medical use of cannabinoids in anxiolytic (stress-reduction) therapies,[2,3,4] but legal statutes on marijuana generally increase the stress levels of millions of cannabis consumers.

Some physicians have recommended cannabis in severe cases such as clinical Post Traumatic Stress Disorder (PTSD).[5] However, the use of an illegal medication to relieve deep anxiety may have limited actual effectiveness. It is predictable that federal prohibition of marijuana will continue to inflict stress on the majority of both recreational and medical cannabis users through harsh penalties and "zero tolerance." Drug war policies remain in force in spite of recommendations by the National Academy of Sciences in the IOM report on medical marijuana: "Recommendation 3: Psychological effects of cannabinoids such as anxiety reduction and sedation, which can influence medical benefits, should be evaluated in clinical trials."[6]

Related sections: *Anxiety Attacks*, page 39; *Incarceration*, page 72; *Paranoia Attacks*, page 90; *Psychoactivity*, page 91.

Stroke and Head Trauma

Stroke and Head Trauma victims frequently suffer a sudden loss of consciousness and sometimes permanent paralysis caused by blood clots within the brain. Stroke is the third leading cause of adult deaths, and there are an estimated 400,000 severe head injury cases per year. In this type of injury, blood flow, and with it oxygen, is cut off to the portion of the brain affected by the blood clot, resulting in brain damage in as little as four minutes. Dr. Raphael Mechoulum, the renowned Israeli scientist who first isolated and synthesized delta-9 tetrahydrocannibinol (THC), designed a synthetic cannabinoid medication that blocks the neural damage caused by oxygen deprivation in cases of stroke, or in cases of traumatic head injury. Remarkably, this new cannabinoid derivative appears to have no toxic effects. The molecule labeled HU-211, which has been called a "wonder drug," may eventually be available in every emergency room around the world.[1] The same drug was labeled dexonabinol in human trials that showed remarkable promise. Patients treated with dexonabinol were found more likely to resume a normal life.[2] Reviewing evidence on the new cannabinoid medication, William Beaver, professor of pharmacology at Georgetown University School of Medicine, was upbeat, saying the drug would be "beyond any doubt the most medically significant use ever made of marijuana."[3] Further studies have discovered that these same properties are also found in other cannabinoids. Pursuing advances of the Israelis, a research team at the US National Institute for Mental Health (NIMH) reported on similar neuron-saving qualities in both THC and another cannabis compound called cannabidiol.[4] The NIMH results suggest that cannabidiol could also become an effective treatment for neurological disorders such as Parkinson's and Alzheimer's diseases.[5] In addition, stroke patients sometimes develop muscle spasms, which are also shown to be relieved by therapeutic cannabis.[6]

Approximately 12 years prior to publication of *The New Prescription*, the author, Martin Martinez, was riding a motorcycle that was struck head-on by an automobile. With a combined speed on impact of 60 miles per hour, the unhelmeted motorcyclist suffered massive skull fractures with resultant cranial swelling and irreparable cranial nerve damage. However, to the amazement of the medical staff and other observers, he did not suffer the cerebral damage typical of such horrendous head trauma. While conducting research on this book, the author eventually concluded that he was spared cognitive damage in this motorcycle crash by a long history of chronic marijuana use. From this anecdotal report, in light of the recent findings by Mechoulum and others, it appears that cannabis may indeed provide an "invisible helmet" of cerebral protection in cases of severe head trauma.

Related sections: *Cerebral Effects*, page 49; *Muscle Spasms*, page 83; *Neuralgia*, page 85.

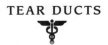

Tear Ducts

Tear Ducts are known to be mildly inhibited by marijuana. The reported reduction in tearing may be related to the "red-eye" symptom common with most users. There are no illnesses or health hazards attributed to this mild side effect.
   Related sections: *Cardiovascular Effects*, page 47.

Testosterone

Testosterone levels were reportedly lowered by "chronic intensive marijuana use" in one 1974 study. These findings have not been substantiated by subsequent research. Two studies concluded that regular administration of cannabinoids reduced testosterone levels in rats, but a review of those studies by Leo Hollister concluded that no significant effect on testosterone or fertility was found. There is no epidemiological evidence that cannabis users are at risk of lowered testosterone levels.
   Related sections: *Fertility*, page 63.

Tolerance

Tolerance, the capacity to consume larger amount of cannabis without adverse effects and with diminishing sensitivity to the psychoactive effects has been established in chronic use. Patients who use copious amounts of cannabis on a daily basis commonly report that they do not experience the stronger psychoactive effects typical of casual use, a finding that has been verified by cognition and psychomotor testing.[1]

The establishment of a tolerance to cannabis was considered evidence of its addictive quality by early researchers. However, as early as 1981 some scientists had concluded that, "Cannabis pharmacology suggests ways of minimizing tolerance and problems."[2] Modern investigations of neuroscience, such as published by the National Institute of Mental Health, indicate that the tolerance factor in cannabis use is entirely different from the tolerance established by classic addictive drugs.[3] While heroin addicts require increasing amounts of the drug to create similar effects, chronic cannabis users discover that marijuana's psychoactive effects actually decrease with increasing amounts and frequency of use.

Tolerance to immune suppression is not well understood, yet has been observed. Australian National Health expert Peter Nelson explains:

> The possibility of tolerance developing to any immunological effects of cannabinoids also makes the human significance of the results of in vitro studies uncertain. If immunological tolerance develops with chronic use, then the possibility of observing even the small effects projected

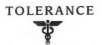

from the in vitro studies would be substantially reduced. Given the large number of cannabinoid effects to which tolerance has been shown to develop, it would not be surprising if this were also true of its immunological effects.[4]

While immunological tolerance is a matter of conjecture, The Institute of Medicine report, Marijuana and Medicine, offered a definitive determination on marijuana tolerance found in cerebral function. In short, according to the IOM: "The brain develops tolerance to cannabinoids."[5]

Related sections: *Addiction*, page 29; *Cerebral Effects*, page 49; *Dependence*, page 57; *Psychoactivity*, page 91; *Psychomotor Skills*, page 94; *Toxicity*, page 114.

Toxicity

Toxicity is virtually nonexistent in natural marijuana. The toxicity levels of cannabis compounds are estimated at 40,000, meaning that a subject would have to ingest 40,000 times the regular dose to induce death. "In layman's terms," according to *The New England Journal of Medicine*, ". . . a smoker would theoretically have to consume nearly 1500 pounds of marijuana within about 15 minutes to induce a lethal response."[1] While that amount of consumption is certainly an impossible feat, in comparison, legal prescription medications cause thousands of deaths per year.[2] Common household drugs are much more lethal than marijuana. For instance, a lethal dose of caffeine is equal to about 100 cups of coffee.[3] In 1972, after reviewing the scientific evidence, the National Commission on Marijuana and Drug Abuse concluded that while marijuana was not entirely safe, its dangers had been grossly overstated.[4] Since then researchers have conducted thousands of studies of humans, animals, and cell cultures. None of those describe any findings dramatically different from those described by the National Commission in 1972.[5] Contaminants, however, are known to be hazardous, especially to those suffering from immune disorders.[6]

Related sections: *Contaminants*, page 54; *Immune Responses*, page 70; *Replacement of Medications*, page 97.

Treating Addiction

Treating Addiction to substances such as heroin, methadone, alcohol, tobacco, and other drugs with a nonaddictive, nontoxic alternative is an effective therapy for some recovering addicts.[1] Trading a physical addiction with serious life-threatening complications for a mild psychological dependence on a harmless substitute may not be the ideal solution; however, cannabis can be a valuable stepping stone to recovery for some addicts.

Research from the University of California, Irvine in April of 1999 showed that anandamide, the natural cannabinoid found in the human brain, inhibits the neurological reactions of dopamine, the brain chemical associated with chemical addiction.[2] As the effects of marijuana include reinforcing the presence of anandamide in the brain, it seems likely that marijuana is not merely a replacement for hard drugs. Cannabis may actually work as an antidote to the neurochemical patterns typical of addiction.

Related sections: *Addiction*, page 29; *Cerebral Effects*, page 49.

Upper Respiratory Infection

Upper Respiratory Infection is an imprecise term referring to almost any infectious disease process involving the upper airway, including nasal passages, pharynx, trachea, or main bronchi. The cause of an upper respiratory infection may be bacterial, fungal, or viral, and is rarely accurately understood.[1]

Although a Canadian report indicates that cannabis is commonly used by North Americans to cure symptoms of the flu and common cold,[2] upper respiratory infection may in fact be a health risk associated with smoking cannabis. Such infections may be in at least some cases related to smoking methods or contamination of marijuana with mold or toxic compounds.

The largest study of its kind in Australia recently focused on 268 long-term marijuana smokers. According to the chief investigator for the Commonwealth Department of Health National Drug Strategy,

> We found nothing startling. We didn't see any evidence of high psychological disturbance among the people. We see very little evidence of health problems except for respiratory problems. [David Reilly, drug and alcohol program manager, Northern Rivers Health Service][3]

The early research of Tashkin et al. and Bloome et al. suggests that chronic cannabis smoking increases the prevalence of bronchitis and may cause an increased susceptibility to bronchogenic carcinoma in chronic cases. However, Huber et al. point out, "there is still no conclusive evidence in man of clinically important pulmonary dysfunction produced by smoking marijuana."[4] Related sections: *Contaminants*, page 54; *Immune Responses*, page 70; *Respiratory Disease*, page 101; *Smoking Methods*, page 107; *Tolerance*, page 113.

Violence

Violence is definitely not triggered by marijuana use, despite the many myths originating in early hemp prohibition propaganda circa 1937. In 1982, the United States National Academy of Science reported in Marijuana and Health,

> Both retrospective and experimental studies in human beings have failed to yield evidence that marijuana use leads to increased aggression. Most of the studies suggest quite the contrary effect. Marijuana appears to have a sedative effect, and it may reduce somewhat the intensity of angry feelings and the probability of aggressive behavior.[1]

Many large sociological studies indicate that violent and sexually aggressive behaviors are directly related to consumption of alcohol.[2] Television is also implicated in violent behaviors in impressionable youths and elderly people.[3] Violent individuals admitted to hospitals are much more likely to have alcohol, cocaine, caffeine, amphetamines, PCP, or other stimulant drugs in their system than marijuana.[4]

Related sections: *Psychoactivity*, page 91; *Stress Reduction*, page 109.

Zelotypia

Zelotypia is a medical term for "monomaniacal zeal in the interest of any project or cause."[1] Medical marijuana patients frequently display a single-minded vehemence for using the natural medicine even when faced with the threat of severe criminal penalties.[2] Such unswerving determination demonstrates the tremendous value of this illegal medicine in improving a patient's quality of life.[3] Similarly, without exception, state laws protecting medical marijuana patients have been won by patients' rights groups that epitomize zelotypia in practice. The nationwide trend of support for medical marijuana laws has developed with extraordinary zeal for the cause.[4]

As of this writing, the medical marijuana controversy rages across America. While critics may refuse to acknowledge the science presented here, brave individuals take heart in the words of Margaret Mead, "Never doubt that a handful of thoughtful committed people can change the world, indeed it is the only thing that ever has."[5]

APPENDICES

Dr. Podrebarac's letter to:

Barry McCaffrey
White House Office of National Drug Control Policy
Executive Office of the President
Washington, DC 20503

Dear Barry McCaffrey,

Please allow me to introduce myself. My name is Francis A. Podrebarac, M.D. I live in Seattle, Washington, and I have been doing extensive study on the benefits of marijuana as medicine. I would like to bring up several points that are not just opinion, but hard evidence that marijuana should be rescheduled for medical use.

The recently released Institute of Medicine (IOM) study on the medical use of marijuana clearly supports rescheduling it for medical use. As you should already know, the IOM report concluded that the active ingredients in marijuana can help fight pain, nausea, anorexia, and anxiety in suffering patients. Hence, marijuana no longer fits the definition of a Schedule I drug. Moreover, the IOM report concluded that marijuana is not a "gateway" drug leading to harder drug use. Rather, alcohol and tobacco appear to be far more notorious for opening doors to harsher, more destructive drug abuse. Marijuana, on the other hand, was reported to be minimally addictive.

APPENDICES

Medical and scientific evidence supporting the rescheduling of marijuana is not new. Before it was prohibited, marijuana was widely prescribed by physicians in the United States and all over the world. In fact, studies during the Nixon administration supported the rescheduling of marijuana.

Marinol was even funded and created by the government in the mid-1980's because marijuana was proving highly beneficial in AIDS patients. However, the federal marijuana access program, Compassionate Use Investigational New Drug Program, was dubiously closed by Health and Human Services (HHS) in 1992. (See Exhibits A and B enclosed: Book by R.C. Randall printed in November 1991 and Los Angeles Times article by Ronald J. Ostrow on January 31,1992.) Both sources point to AIDS discrimination as the reason it was closed. The closing of the Compassionate Use IND Program was illegal because it violated Title 3 of the Americas with Disabilities Act of 1990. Furthermore, HHS continuing to provide access to a few patients, even to this day, is illegal because they are providing legal medicinal marijuana access to a select few while denying access to the majority of suffering patients who might also benefit from medical use of marijuana.

The New England Journal of Medicine (NEJM) also supports the rescheduling of marijuana for medical use. The editor-in-chief, Jerome P. Kassirer, M.D., suggested that a federal policy prohibiting physicians from helping their suffering patients by suggesting that they use marijuana is "misguided, heavy-handed, and inhumane." He recommended that marijuana be rescheduled and be made available by prescription and correctly noted that the DEA recommended marijuana be rescheduled in September 1998, after 2 years of extensive hearings into the matter. (See January 30, 1997, NEJM article enclosed as Exhibit C. A second article in the NEJM supporting the rescheduling of marijuana, dated August 7, 1997, by George J. Annas, J.D, M.P.H., is also enclosed as Exhibit D.)

As you can see from the evidence that I have provided, there is a great injustice being done to Americans who are suffering and could benefit from using marijuana as medicine. I would be more than happy to testify before your committee, at any time, because I believe in truth in medical research and medical practice. I have seen what kind of a difference marijuana can make in the lives of people who are truly suffering, and I urge you, on their behalf, to please immediately reschedule marijuana and treat it accordingly. Our country doesn't need 50 different marijuana laws in 50 different states. Doctors and patients are not the enemy in the war on drugs, nor do we belong in the crossfire. You are the one who can turn this around and provide relief from suffering to millions of people across the nation.

Thank you so much for your time.

Sincerely,

Francis A. Podrebarac, M.D.

Graduate University of Kansas School of Medicine—1988
Diplomat American Board of Psychiatry and Neurology—1994
Diplomat Added Qualifications Exam Geriatric Psychiatry—1996

APPENDICES

Letter to Dr. Podrebarac from:

EXECUTIVE OFFICE OF THE PRESIDENT
OFFICE OF NATIONAL DRUG CONTROL POLICY
Washington, D.C. 20503
May 3. 1999

Dr. Francis A. Podrebarac, M.D.
Seattle, Washington

Dear Dr. Podrebarac:

It was good to talk to you in March. Director McCaffrey shared you letter of April 14th in which you offered several points for ONDCP consideration in light of the Institute of Medicine (IOM) study Marijuana and Medicine: Assessing the Science Base and asked me to respond.

In our view, this IOM study is the most comprehensive summary and analysis of what is known about the use of marijuana and its constituent cannabinoids for medicinal purposes, marijuana's mechanism of action, peer-reviewed literature on the uses of marijuana, and costs associated with various forms of the component chemical compounds in marijuana. We believe the following points must be taken into account as a result of the IOM study's conclusions and recommendations:

There is little future for smoked marijuana as a medically approved medication. As the study emphasizes, existing scientific evidence already indicates that smoking cannabis—or smoking any plant material—is carcinogenic and toxic to the lungs. Modern medicine identifies and then synthesizes active components in plants with potential medical benefits to allow for the most safe and effective scientific uses.

Research into the physiological effects of marijuana and its constituent cannabinoids should continue. The identification of cannabinoid receptors in the brain provides a sound basis for further research. The report notes cannabinoid-based medicines may have the potential to contribute to symptom management programs for a number of afflictions and diseases.

Bonafide clinical trials of smoked marijuana must be designed with rigor and conducted with care. Genuine clinical research in the specific areas recommended by the IOM study should be facilitated. Such clinical trial should facilitate the development of an inhaler or alternate rapid-onset delivery system for THC or other cannabinoid drugs.

Continue strict regulation of cannabis is essential. It is absolutely essential that we have strict regulation of this drug. We need to be sure that as we examine cannabinoid-based drugs for possible medical benefit that we do not contribute to increased abuse of this psychoactive substance.

We are hopeful that as a result of the IOM study, the discussion of the medical efficacy and safety of cannabinoids can take place within the context of medicine and science. Indeed, we are working closely with the Department of Health and Human Services to encourage bonafide clinical research of cannabinoids and to insure appropriate medical access to drugs and substances that are deemed safe and effective for medical use in treatment. Thank you again for sharing your views with us.

Best wishes,

Francis X. Kinney
Director of Strategy

Institute of Medicine Executive Summary

MARIJUANA AND MEDICINE

Assessing the Science Base

Janet E. Joy, Stanley J. Watson, Jr., and
John A. Benson, Jr., Editors

NATIONAL ACADEMY PRESS
Washington D.C., 1999

Executive Summary

Public opinion on the medical value of marijuana has been sharply divided. Some dismiss medical marijuana as a hoax that exploits our natural compassion for the sick; others claim it is a uniquely soothing medicine that has been withheld from patients through regulations based on false claims. Proponents of both views cite "scientific evidence" to support their views and have expressed those views at the ballot box in recent state elections. In January 1997, the White House Office of National Drug Control Policy (ONDCP) asked the Institute of Medicine (IOM) to conduct a review of the scientific evidence to assess the potential health benefits and risks of marijuana and its constituent cannabinoids (see the Statement of Task on page 9). That review began in August 1997 and culminates with this report.

The ONDCP request came in the wake of state "medical marijuana" initiatives. In November 1996, voters in California and Arizona passed referenda designed to permit the use of marijuana as medicine. Although Arizona's referendum was invalidated five months later, the referenda galvanized a national response. In November 1998, voters in six states (Alaska, Arizona, Colorado, Nevada, Oregon, and Washington) passed ballot initiatives in support of medical marijuana. (The Colorado vote will not count, however, because after the vote was taken a court ruling determined there had not been enough valid signatures to place the initiative on the ballot.)

Can marijuana relieve health problems? Is it safe for medical use? Those straightforward questions are embedded in a web of social concerns, most of which lie outside the scope of this report. Controversies concerning the nonmedical use of marijuana spill over into the medical marijuana debate and obscure the real state of scientific knowledge. In contrast with the many disagreements bearing on social issues, the study team found substantial consensus among experts in the relevant disciplines on the scientific evidence about potential medical uses of marijuana.

This report summarizes and analyzes what is known about the medical use of marijuana; it emphasizes evidence-based medicine (derived from knowledge and experience informed by rigorous scientific analysis), as opposed to belief-based medicine (derived from judgment, intuition, and beliefs untested by rigorous science).

Throughout this report, *marijuana* refers to unpurified plant substances, including leaves or flower tops whether consumed by ingestion or smoking. References to the "effects of marijuana" should be understood to include the composite effects of its various components; that is, the effects of tetrahydrocannabinol (THC), which is the primary psychoactive ingredient in marijuana, are included among its effects, but not all the effects of marijuana are necessarily due to THC. *Cannabinoids* are the group of compounds related to THC, whether found in the marijuana plant, in animals, or synthesized in chemistry laboratories.

Three focal concerns in evaluating the medical use of marijuana are:

1. Evaluation of the effects of isolated cannabinoids;
2. Evaluation of the risks associated with the medical use of marijuana; and
3. Evaluation of the use of smoked marijuana.

EFFECTS OF ISOLATED CANNABINOIDS

Cannabinoid Biology

Much has been learned since the 1982 IOM report Marijuana and Health. Although it was clear then that most of the effects of marijuana were due to its actions on the brain, there was little infor-

were affected by THC, or even what general areas of the brain were most affected by THC. In addition, too little was known about cannabinoid physiology to offer any   scientific insights into the harmful or therapeutic effects of marijuana. That all changed with the identification and characterization of cannabinoid receptors in the 1980s and 1990s. During the past 16 years, science has advanced greatly and can tell us much more about the potential medical benefits of cannabinoids.

Conclusion: At this point, our knowledge about the biology of marijuana and cannabinoids allows us to make some general conclusions:

- Cannabinoids likely have a natural role in pain modulation, control of movement, and memory.
- The natural role of cannabinoids in immune systems is likely multi-faceted and remains unclear.
- The brain develops tolerance to cannabinoids.
- Animal research demonstrates the potential for dependence, but this potential is observed under a narrower range of conditions than with benzodiazepines, opiates, cocaine, or nicotine.
- Withdrawal symptoms can be observed in animals but appear to be mild compared to opiates or benzdiazepines, such as diazepam (Valium).

Conclusion: The different cannabinoid receptor types found in the body appear to play different roles in normal human physiology. In addition, some effects of cannabinoids appear to be independent of those receptors. The variety of mechanisms through which cannabinoids can influence human physiology underlies the variety of potential therapeutic uses for drugs that might act selectively on different cannabinoid systems.

Recommendation 1: Research should continue into the physiological effects of synthetic and plant-derived cannabinoids and the natural function of cannabinoids found in the body. Because different cannabinoids appear to have different effects, cannabinoid research should include, but not be restricted to, effects attributable to THC alone.

APPENDICES

Efficacy of Cannabinoid Drugs

The accumulated data indicate a potential therapeutic value for cannabinoid drugs, particularly for symptoms such as pain relief, control of nausea and vomiting, and appetite stimulation. The therapeutic effects of cannabinoids are best established for THC, which is generally one of the two most abundant of the cannabinoids in marijuana. (Cannabidiol is generally the other most abundant cannabinoid.)

The effects of cannabinoids on the symptoms studied are generally modest, and in most cases there are more effective medications. However, people vary in their responses to medications, and there will likely always be a subpopulation of patients who do not respond well to other medications. The combination of cannabinoid drug effects (anxiety reduction, appetite stimulation, nausea reduction, and pain relief) suggests that cannabinoids would be moderately well suited for particular conditions, such as chemotherapy-induced nausea and vomiting and AIDS wasting.

Defined substances, such as purified cannabinoid compounds, are preferable to plant products, which are of variable and uncertain composition. Use of defined cannabinoids permits a more precise evaluation of their effects, whether in combination or alone. Medications that can maximize the desired effects of cannabinoids and minimize the undesired effects can very likely be identified.

Although most scientists who study cannabinoids agree that the pathways to cannabinoid drug development are clearly marked, there is no guarantee that the fruits of scientific research will be made available to the public for medical use. Cannabinoid-based drugs will only become available if public investment in cannabinoid drug research is sustained and if there is enough incentive for private enterprise to develop and market such drugs.

Conclusion: Scientific data indicate the potential therapeutic value of cannabinoid drugs, primarily THC, for pain relief, control of nausea and vomiting, and appetite stimulation; smoked marijuana, however, is a crude THC delivery system that also delivers harmful substances.

Recommendation 2: Clinical trials of cannabinoid drugs for symptom management should be conducted with the goal of developing rapid-onset, reliable, and safe delivery systems.

127

Influence of Psychological Effects on Therapeutic Effects

The psychological effects of THC and similar cannabinoids pose three issues for the therapeutic use of cannabinoid drugs. First, for some patients—particularly older patients with no previous marijuana experience—the psychological effects are disturbing. Those patients report experiencing unpleasant feelings and disorientation after being treated with THC, generally more severe for oral THC than for smoked marijuana. Second, for conditions such as movement disorders or nausea, in which anxiety exacerbates the symptoms, the antianxiety effects of cannabinoid drugs can influence symptoms indirectly. This can be beneficial or can create false impressions of the drug effect. Third, for cases in which symptoms are multifaceted, the combination of THC effects might provide a form of adjunctive therapy; for example, AIDS wasting patients would likely benefit from a medication that simultaneously reduces anxiety, pain, and nausea while stimulating appetite.

Conclusion: The psychological effects of cannabinoids, such as anxiety reduction, sedation, and euphoria can influence their potential therapeutic value. Those effects are potentially undesirable for certain patients and situations and beneficial for others. In addition, psychological effects can complicate the interpretation of other aspects of the drug's effect.

Recommendation 3: Psychological effects of cannabinoids such as anxiety reduction and sedation, which can influence medical benefits, should be evaluated in clinical trials.

RISKS ASSOCIATED WITH MEDICAL USE OF MARIJUANA

Physiological Risks

Marijuana is not a completely benign substance. It is a powerful drug with a variety of effects. However, except for the harms associated with smoking, the adverse effects of marijuana use are within the range of effects tolerated for other medications. The harmful effects to individuals from the perspective of possible medical use of marijuana are not necessarily the same as the harmful physical effects of drug abuse. When interpreting studies purporting to show the harmful effects of marijuana, it is important to keep in mind that the majority of those studies are based on smoked marijuana, and cannabinoid effects cannot be separated from the effects of inhaling smoke from burning plant material and contaminants. For most people the primary adverse effect of acute marijuana use is diminished psychomotor performance. It is, therefore, inadvisable to operate any vehicle or potentially dangerous equipment while under the influence of marijuana, THC, or any cannabinoid drug with comparable effects. In addition, a minority of marijuana users experience dysphoria, or unpleasant feelings. Finally, the short-term immunosuppressive effects are not well established but, if they exist, are not likely great enough to preclude a legitimate medical use.

The chronic effects of marijuana are of greater concern for medical use and fall into two categories: the effects of chronic smoking and the effects of THC. Marijuana smoking is associated with abnormalities of cells lining the human respiratory tract. Marijuana smoke, like tobacco smoke, is associated with increased risk of cancer, lung damage, and poor pregnancy outcomes. Although cellular, genetic, and human studies all suggest that marijuana smoke is an important risk factor for the development of respiratory cancer, proof that habitual marijuana smoking does or does not cause cancer awaits the results of well-designed studies.

Conclusion: Numerous studies suggest that marijuana smoke is an important risk factor in the development of respiratory disease.

Recommendation 4: Studies to define the individual health risks of smoking marijuana should be conducted, particularly among populations in which marijuana use is prevalent.

Marijuana Dependence and Withdrawal

A second concern associated with chronic marijuana use is dependence on the psychoactive effects of THC. Although few marijuana users develop dependence, some do. Risk factors for marijuana dependence are similar to those for other forms of substance abuse. In particular, anti-social person-ality and conduct disorders are

Conclusion: A distinctive marijuana withdrawal syndrome has been identified, but it is mild and short lived. The syndrome includes restlessness, irritability, mild agitation, insomnia, sleep disturbance, nausea, and cramping.

Marijuana as a "Gateway" Drug

Patterns in progression of drug use from adolescence to adulthood are strikingly regular. Because it is the most widely used illicit drug, marijuana is predictably the first illicit drug most people encounter. Not surprisingly, most users of other illicit drugs have used marijuana first. In fact, most drug users begin with alcohol and nicotine before marijuana—usually before they are of legal age.

In the sense that marijuana use typically precedes rather than follows initiation of other illicit drug use, it is indeed a "gateway" drug. But because underage smoking and alcohol use typically precede marijuana use, marijuana is not the most common, and is rarely the first, "gateway" to illicit drug use. There is no conclusive evidence that the drug effects of marijuana are causally linked to the subsequent abuse of other illicit drugs. An important caution is that data on drug use progression cannot be assumed to apply to the use of drugs for medical purposes. It does not follow from those data that if marijuana were available by prescription for medical use, the pattern of drug use would remain the same as seen in illicit use.

Finally, there is a broad social concern that sanctioning the medical use of marijuana might increase its use among the general population. At this point there are no convincing data to support this concern. The existing data are consistent with the idea that this would not be a problem if the medical use of marijuana were as closely regulated as other medications with abuse potential.

Conclusion: Present data on drug use progression neither support nor refute the suggestion that medical availability would increase drug abuse. However, this question is beyond the issues normally considered for medical uses of drugs and should not be a factor in evaluating the therapeutic potential of marijuana or cannabinoids.

USE OF SMOKED MARIJUANA

Because of the health risks associated with smoking, smoked marijuana should generally not be recommended for long-term medical use. Nonetheless, for certain patients, such as the terminally ill or those with debilitating symptoms, the long-term risks are not of great concern. Further, despite the legal, social, and health problems associated with smoking marijuana, it is widely used by certain patient groups.

Recommendation 5: Clinical trials of marijuana use for medical purposes should be conducted under the following limited circumstances: trials should involve only   short-term marijuana use (less than six months), should be conducted in patients with conditions for which there is reasonable expectation of efficacy, should be approved by institutional review boards, and should collect data about efficacy.

The goal of clinical trials of smoked marijuana would not be to develop marijuana as a licensed drug but rather to serve as a first step toward the possible development of nonsmoked rapid-onset cannabinoid delivery systems. However, it will likely be many years before a safe and effective cannabinoid delivery system, such as an inhaler, is available for patients. In the meantime there are patients with debilitating symptoms for whom smoked marijuana might provide relief. The use of smoked marijuana for those patients should weigh both the expected efficacy of marijuana and ethical issues in patient care, including providing information about the known and suspected risks of smoked marijuana use.

Recommendation 6: Short-term use of smoked marijuana (less than six months) for patients with debilitating symptoms (such as intractable pain or vomiting) must meet the following conditions:
• failure of all approved medications to provide relief has been documented,
• the symptoms can reasonably be expected to be relieved by rapid-onset cannabinoid drugs,

- such treatment is administered under medical supervision in a manner that allows for assessment of treatment effectiveness, and
- involves an oversight strategy comparable to an institutional review board process that could provide guidance within 24 hours of a submission by a physician to provide marijuana to a patient for a specified use.

Until a nonsmoked rapid-onset cannabinoid drug delivery system becomes available, we acknowledge that there is no clear alternative for people suffering from chronic conditions that might be relieved by smoking marijuana, such as pain or AIDS wasting. One possible approach is to treat patients as n-of-1 clinical trials (single-patient trials), in which patients are fully informed of their status as experimental subjects using a harmful drug delivery system and in which their condition is closely monitored and documented under medical supervision, thereby increasing the knowledge base of the risks and benefits of marijuana use under such conditions.

NOTES

ACQUIRED IMMUNE DEFICIENCY SYNDROME

1. "UN says HIV more widespread than thought." Associated Press, November 26, 1997
2. "Study shows first downturn in AIDS." Associated Press, September 19, 1997
3. Jacobson, "US Deaths from AIDS dropped 12% in period, study finds." *Dallas Morning Star*, February 28, 1998
4. "CDC says a third of HIV cases untreated." Associated Press, September 26, 1997
5. "AIDS cases up dramatically among Americans 50 and up." *Newsday*, January 23, 1998
6. ABC Evening News, July 11, 1998
7. "Study shows first downturn in AIDS," Associated Press, September 19, 1997
8. Palella et al., "Declining morbidity and mortality among patients with advanced human immunodeficiency virus." *New England Journal of Medicine*, Vol. 338, No. 13, p. 853, March 26, 1998
9. "AIDS drugs fail many." *Seattle Times*, September 30 1997
10. ACT UP, www.actupgg.org
11. "New lifesaving drugs explored as possible culprit." Associated Press, May 14, 1998
12. Conversations with Dr. Francis Podrebarac, MD, 1998-1999
13. Laino, "Waiting to inhale: Hemp for health?" *MSNBC News*, Spring 1998
14. McWilliams, "Medical marijuana and me." Source: Grinspoon, The Forbidden Medicine Website, www.rxmarihuana.com
15. Podrebarac, *op. cit.*
16. McWilliams, Testimony before the California Senate Medical Marijuana Distribution Summit, May 26, 1998
17. Abrams, Lindesmith Center Lecture, San Francisco, May 17, 1999
18. Institute of Medicine, *Marijuana and Medicine: Assessing the Science Base.* Washington, DC: National Academy Press, 1999
19. Podrebarac, *op. cit.*
20. Abrams, *op. cit.*
21. Kaslow et al., *World Health Organization Project on Health Implications of Cannabis Use*

22. *California NORML Reports*, Vol. 21, No. 3, October, 1997
23. Latimer, "Highwitness news." *High Times,* No. 270, p. 30, February, 1998
24. Abrams, *op. cit.*
25. "NIH panelists agree: marijuana is safe and effective medicine." *MPP News,* Marijuana Policy Project, August 4, 1997, www.mpp.org
26. Institute of Medicine, *op. cit.*
27. "Federal report reignites medical marijuana debate." CNN, March 17, 1999
28. "Medicinal marijuana briefing paper 1997-98." *Marijuana Policy Project,* 1998, www.mpp.org
29. "Feds OK Marijuana Research." *Los Angeles Times,* May 21, 1999
30. Abrams, *op. cit.*
31. "Federal report reignites medical marijuana debate." CNN, March 17, 1999
32. Doblin and Kleiman, "Marijuana as anti-emetic medicine: A survey of oncologists experiences and attitudes." *Journal of Clinical Oncology,* Vol. 9, pp. 1314-1319, 1991
33. Robson, "Cannabis as medicine: time for the phoenix to rise?" *British Medical Journal,* Vol. 316, No. 7137, p. 1034(2), 1998
34. "CMA backs removal of marijuana from Schedule I prohibitive status." *NORML News,* May 28, 1998
35. "NY State Legislator and head of NY Hospital's Department of Public Health Supports medical marijuana." Source: Cowen, www.marijuananews.com, January 1998
36. Oakland City Council Resolutions on Medical Marijuana, June 1998
37. Robson, *op. cit.*
38. Robson, *op. cit.*
39. Statement of the British Medical Association. February 1994
40. (All organizations not individually noted) Medical Groups' Endorsements. *NORML News*
41. www.mpp.org/science.html#12
42. McWilliams, "In the war on drugs, a Red Cross is just another target." www.petertrial.com

ADDICTION

1. Taber's Cyclopedic Medical Dictionary. Philadelphia: F. A. Davis Company, 1987
2. "US Study: Marijuana is addictive." Reuters, March 31, 1998
3. "New Scientist special report on marijuana." New Scientist, February 21, 1998
4. "US Study: Marijuana is addictive." *op. cit.*
5. Institute of Medicine, Marijuana and Medicine: Assessing the Science Base. Washington, DC: National Academy Press, 1999
6. "Similar effects found for pot, harder drugs." Maugh, Los Angeles Times, June 27, 1997
7. Castaneda et al., "THC does not affect striatal dopamine release: microdialysis in freely moving rats." 1991
8. Gifford, Gardner, and Ashby, "The effects of intravenous administration of delta-9-tetrahydrocannabinol on the activity of A10 dopamine neurons recorded in vivo in anesthetized rats." Neuropsychopharmacology Vol. 36, No. 2, pp. 96-99, 1997

NOTES

9. "The July 1995 Gettman/High Times petition to repeal marijuana prohibition: An extensive review of relevant legal and scientific findings." Source: www.hightimes.com/ht/new/petition/jgpetition/index.html

10. "Researchers watch dopamine changes in brain of video game players." Associated Press, May 21, 1998

11. Nelson, "A Critical Review of the Research Literature Concerning Some Biological and Psychological Effects of Cannabis." Advisory Committee on Illicit Drugs, Cannabis and the law in Queensland, pp. 113-152, Source: Schaffer Library of Drug Policy, www.druglibrary.org

12. Piomelli, "Functional role of high-affinity anandamide transport, as revealed by selective inhibition." Science, Vol. 277, No. 5329, p. 1094(4), August 22, 1997

13. Gettman, op. cit., See also: Gettman, "Marijuana and the human brain." High Times, March 1995

14. "Chocolate and Cannabinol." The Washington Post, August 26, 1996

15. Stein, "Bits and Pieces." Geriatric Psychiatry News, Issue 3, No. 7, June/July 1999

16. U.S. Congress OTA, 1993

17. Grinspoon, Bakalar, Zimmer, and Morgan, "Marijuana addiction." Science, Vol. 277, p. 749, August 8, 1997

18. Annas, "Reefer Madness—The federal response to California's medical-marijuana law." The New England Journal of Medicine, Vol. 337, No. 6, August 7, 1997

19. Zimmer and Morgan, Marijuana Myths: Marijuana Facts. New York: The Lindesmith Center, 1997

20. U.S. Code Congressional and Administrative News, 1970

21. Institute of Medicine, Marijuana and Medicine: Assessing the Science Base. Washington, DC: National Academy Press, 1999

22. "DEA refers marijuana rescheduling petition to HHS." The Law Offices of Michael Kennedy, NY, 1998

23. "Official report backs medical use of marijuana." Reuters, March 17, 1999

ANALGESIA

1. Doctor urges war on pain, more use of opium-based drugs." Miami Herald, January 29, 1998

2. Stolberg, "Study Finds Elderly Receive Little Pain Treatment in Nursing Homes." June 17, 1998

3. Doctor urges war on pain, more use of opium-based drugs." Miami Herald, January 29, 1998

4. "Researchers say many cancer patients suffer needless pain." Associated Press, June 17, 1998

5. Drug Enforcement Administration, "Statement of policy for the use and handling of controlled bstances in the treatment of pain." 1998

6. Kassirer, "Federal foolishness and marijuana." Editorial, The New England Journal of Medicine, January 30, 1997

7. Mikuriya, Marijuana Medical Papers: 1839-1972. Oakland: Medi-comp Press, 1973

8. Grinspoon, Marijuana Reconsidered. 3rd ed. San Francisco: Quick American Archives, 1971

9. Noyes and Baram, "Cannabis analgesia." Comprehensive Psychiatry, Vol. 15, No. 6, 1974

10. Beltramo and Piomelli, "Functional role of high-affinity anandamide transport, as revealed by selective inhibition." Science, Vol. 277, No. 5329, p1094(4), 1997

11. Formukong, Evans, and Evans, "Analgesic and anti-inflammatory activity of constituents of cannabis sativa L." *Inflammation,* Vol. 12, No. 4, pp. 361-371, 1988

12. Maurer, Henn, Dittrich, and Hofmann, "Delta-9-tetrahydrocannabinol shows
   antispastic and analgesic effects in a single case double-blind trial." *European
   Archive of Psychiatry and Neurological Science,* Vol. 240, No. 1, pp. 1-4, 1990

13. "Cannabidiol: Wonder drug of the 21st century?" Source: Schaffer Library of Drug
   Policy, www.druglibrary.org

14. "Pre-clinical Studies show CT-3 Reduces chronic and acute inflammation and
   reduces destruction of joints." BW HealthWire, January 1998

15. Portyansky, *Plant of a Thousand Uses (marijuana).* Medical Economics Publishing,
   1998, Electronic Collection: A20409468

16. "Medical marijuana: Doing the science." *Synapse,* 1998,
   www.itsa.ucsf.edu/synapse/

17. Symposium Syllabus: *Functional Role of Cannabinoid Receptors.* Press
   Conference, August 26, 1998, Source: Medical Marijuana Magazine,
   www.marijuanamagazine.com

18. "Study reveals pot chemicals can relieve serious pain." *Los Angeles Times,*
   October 27, 1998

19. *Ibid.*

20. Morin, "Research into cannabinoids provides evidence that the use of marijuana
   to treat pain and nausea should not be so easily dismissed." May 1998, Source:
   Morin@Brown.edu

21. Cowen, "Science journal reports that cannabinoid receptors located outside the
   brain and spine are affected when the skin or flesh is cut or hurt." July 16, 1998,
   www.marijuananews.com

22. Widener, "Study: Marijuana, morphine work on same area of brain." *The Seattle
   Times,* September 25, 1998

23. "Diagnosis: Smoke Pot to Relieve Pain." *The University of Washington Daily,*
   May 1997

24. Abrams, Lindesmith Center Lecture, San Francisco, May 17, 1999

25. Holdcroft et al., "Pain relief with oral cannabinoids in familial Mediterranean
   fever." *Anaesthesia,* Vol. 52, No. 5, pp. 483-486, May 1997

26. *San Francisco Chronicle, San Francisco Examiner,* Associated Press, May 1998

27. Institute of Medicine, *Marijuana and Medicine: Assessing the Science Base.*
   Washington DC: National Academy Press, 1999

ANTIBIOTIC

1. Grinspoon, *Marijuana Reconsidered.* 3rd ed. San Francisco: Quick American
   Archives, 1971

ANTIMOTIVATIONAL SYNDROME

1. Kolansky and Moore, 1971, Millman and Sbriglio, 1986, from: World Health
   Organization Project on Health Implications of Cannabis Use. 1997

2. Dornbush, 1974, Negrete, 1983, Hollister, "Health aspects of marijuana."
   Pharmacological Review, Vol. 38, No. 1, 1986

3. World Health Organization Project on Health Implications of Cannabis Use. 1997

4. American Civil Liberties Union statement on marijuana prohibition. May 1998

5. Grinspoon, Marijuana Reconsidered. 3rd ed. San Francisco: Quick American
   Archives, 1971

NOTES

6. Schaeffer, Andrysiak, and Ungerleider, "Cognition and long term use of ganja."
   Science, Vol. 213, pp. 465-466, July 24, 1981

ARTHRITIS

1. "Pot chemical can relieve serious pain." *Los Angeles Times*, August 27, 1998
2. Formukong, Evans, and Evans, "Analgesic and anti-inflammatory activity of constituents of cannabis sativa L." *Inflammation*, Vol. 12, No. 4 p. 361-371, 1988
3. Hollister, "Health Aspects of Marijuana." *Pharmacological Review*, Vol. 38, No. 1, 1986
4. Symposium Syllabus: *Functional Role of Cannabinoid Receptors*. August 26, 1998
5. Institute of Medicine, *Marijuana and Medicine: Assessing the Science Base*.
   Washington DC: National Academy Press, 1999

ASTHMA

1. Grinspoon, "Marijuana and asthma." The Forbidden Medicine Website,
   www.rxmarihuana.com
2. National Academy of Science, 1982
3. "Therapeutic possibilities in cannabinoids," Editorial, *The Lancet*, pp. 667-669,
   March 22, 1975
4. Tashkin, Shapiro, Lee, and Harper, "Effects of smoked marijuana in experimentally induced asthma." *American Review of Respiratory Disease*, Vol. 112, 1975
5. Grinspoon and Bakalar, *Marijuana: The Forbidden Medicine*. New Haven: Yale
   University Press, 1997
6. Letters, *High Times*, No. 273, May, 1998
7. Institute of Medicine, *Marijuana and Medicine: Assessing the Science Base*.
   Washington DC: National Academy Press, 1999
8. Geiringer, "An overview of the human research studies on medical use of marijuana." CANORML, 1994, www.norml.org/canorml/

CANCER

1. Poster, Penta, Bruno, and Macdonald, "Delta-9-tetrahydrocannabinol in clinical
   oncology." *Journal of the American Medical Association*, Vol. 245, No. 20, pp.
   2047-2051, May 22, 1988
2. Orr, Mckernan, and Bloome, "Anti-emetic effect of tetrahydrocannabinol compared with placebo and prochlorperazine in chemotherapy-associated nausea
   and emisis." *Archives of Internal Medicine*, Vol. 140, No. 11, pp. 1431-1433,
   November 1980
3. Williams, Boulton, de Pemberton, and Whitehouse, "Antiemetics for patients
   treated with antitumor chemotherapy." *Cancer Clinical Trials*, Vol. 3, No. 4, pp.
   363-367, 1980
4. Ekert, Waters, Jurk, Mobilia, and Loughnan, "Amelioration of cancer chemotherapy-induced nausea and vomiting by delta-9-tetrahydrocannabinol." *Medical
   Journal of Australia*, Vol. 2, No. 12, pp. 657-659, December 15, 1979
5. Williams, Boulton, de Pemberton, and Whitehouse, *op. cit.*
6. "American Medical Association House of Delegates Report." December 9, 1997
7. Seeley, *Town Meeting*. KOMO TV 4 in Seattle, March 9, 1997
8. National Cancer Institute, *Marijuana Use in Supportive Care for Cancer Patients*.
   Cancer Information Service, September 1997, Source: http://cancernet.nci/

NOTES

9. Vinciguerra, Moore, and Brennen, "Inhalation of marijuana as an anti-emetic for chemotherapy." *New York State Journal of Medicine*, Vol. 88, pp. 525-527, 1988

10. NORML News. February 13, 1998, www.norml.org

11. "NIH panelists agree: Marijuana is safe and effective medicine." *MPP News,* Marijuana Policy Project, August 4, 1997, www.mpp.org

12. Abrams, Lindesmith Center Lecture, San Francisco, May 17, 1999

13. Abrahamov, Abrahamov, and Mechoulam, "An efficient new cannabinoid anti-emetic in pediatric oncology." The Brettler Center for Medical Research, Hebrew University, Jerusalem, 1995

14. Doblin and Kleiman, "Marijuana as anti-emetic medicine: A survey of oncologists experiences and attitudes." *Journal of Clinical Oncology*, Vol. 9, pp. 1314-1319, 1991

15. Sallen, Zinburg, and Frei, "Anti-emetic effects of Delta-9 THC in patients receiving cancer chemotherapy." *New England Journal of Medicine*, Vol. 296, No. 16, 1975

16. Gieringer, "Review of Human Studies on Medical Use of Marijuana." 1994, CANORML, www.norml.org/canorml/

17. Letter from American Cancer Society to CA Senator Vasconcellos, July 25, 1997

18. Conversations with Ralph Seely and others, 1997-1998

19. Noyes, Brunk, Baram, and Canter, "Analgesic effect of delta-9-tetrahydro-cannabinol." *Journal of Clinical Pharmacology*, Vol. 2, No. 3, pp. 139-143, February 15, 1975

20. Statement of Dr. Richard Cohen, Consulting Medical Oncologist, California-Pacific Medical Center, San Francisco. Source: Californians for Medical Rights

21. Institute of Medicine, *Marijuana and Medicine: Assessing the Science Base.* Washington DC: National Academy Press, 1999

22. Grinspoon and Bakalar, *Medical Uses of Illicit Drugs*, 1997

23. Bertrand, Affidavit before Ontario Court (Canada) in the case of Christopher Clay, Source: www.hempnation.com/challenge/bertrand.html

24. Abrams, *op. cit.*

25. James, "Medical marijuana: Unpublished federal study found THC treated rats lived longer, had fewer cancers." *AIDS Treatment News*, January 17, 1997

26. Knox, "Study may undercut marijuana opponents: Report says THC did not cause cancer." *Boston Globe*, January 30, 1997

27. Abrams, *op. cit.*

28. Hollister, "Health Aspects of Marijuana." *Pharmacological Review*, Vol. 38, No. 1, 1986

29. Institute of Medicine, *op. cit.*

30. Hollister, *op. cit.*

CARDIOVASCULAR EFFECTS

1. "The health and psychological consequences of cannabis use." Chapter 6, National Drug Strategy Monograph No. 25, Australia

2. Nelson, "A critical review of the research literature concerning some biological and psychological effects of cannabis." Advisory Committee on Illicit Drugs, Cannabis and the Law in Queensland: Criminal Justice Commission of Queensland, Australia, 1993

3. Nelson, op. cit.

4. Nelson, op. cit.

NOTES

5.   Avakian, Horvath, Michael, and Jacobs, "Effects of marijuana on cardio-respiratory responses to submaximal exercise." *Clinical Pharmacological Therapeutics*, Vol. 6, pp. 777-781, 1979

6.   World Health Organization Project on Health Implications of Cannabis Use, 1997

7.   Hollister, "Health Aspects of Marijuana." *Pharmacological Review*, Vol. 38, No. 1, 1986

8.   "The health and psychological consequences of cannabis use." Chapter 6, National Drug Strategy Monograph No. 25, Australia

9.   Ibid.

10.   Mikuriya, Marijuana Medical Handbook, Source: Schaffer Library of Drug Policy, www.druglibrary.org

CEREBRAL EFFECTS

1.   Gettman, "Drug Abuse, Cannabis and the Brain." High Times, 1997, www.hightimes.com, See also: Gettman, 1995

2.   Maugh, "Similar effects found for pot, harder drugs." *Los Angeles Times*: Science Focus, June 27, 1997

3.   Gifford, Gardner, and Ashby, "The effects of intravenous administration of delta-9-tetrahydrocannabinol on the activity of A10 dopamine neurons recorded in vivo in anesthetized rats." *Neuropsychopharmacology*, Vol. 36, No. 2, pp. 96-99, 1997

4.   Finn, "Cannabinoid Investigations Entering The Mainstream." *The Scientist*, Vol. 12, No. 3, pp. 1-8, February 2, 1998

5.   Beltramo and Piomelli, "Functional role of high-affinity anandamide transport, as revealed by selective inhibition," *Science*, Vol. 277, No. 5329, p. 1094(4), August 22, 1997

6.   Mathew, Wilson, Coleman, Turkington, and DeGrado, "Marijuana intoxication and brain activation in marijuana smokers." *Life Science*, Vol. 60, No. 23, pp. 2075-2089, 1997

7.   Devane et al., *Science*, Vol. 258, pp. 1946-1949, 1992

8.   Axelrod, "Enzymatic synthesis of anandamide, an endogenous ligand for the cannabinoid receptor, by brain membranes." Laboratory of Cell Biology, National Institute of Mental Health, Bethesda MD, 1997

9.   Fackelmann, "Marijuana and the brain: scientists discover the brain's own THC." *Science News*, Vol. 143, No. 6, p. 88, February 6, 1993

10.   Zimmer and Morgan, *Marijuana Myths: Marijuana Facts*. New York: The Lindesmith Center, 1997

11.   Aigner, "Delta-9 tetrahydrocannabinol impairs visual recognition memory but not discrimination learning in rhesus monkeys." *Psychopharmacology*, Vol. 95, No. 4, pp. 507-511, 1988

12.   Institute of Medicine, *Marijuana and Medicine: Assessing the Science Base*. Washington DC: National Academy Press, 1999

13.   "Cannabis: Look, Listen, Learn," *Independent* (UK), cannabis@independentco.org, 1998, Source: Media Awareness Project, www.mapinc.org

14.   "Planet Science: Marijuana special report." *New Scientist*, February 21, 1998

15.   Schaeffer, Andrysiak, and Ungerleider, "Cognition and long term use of ganja." *Science*, Vol. 213, pp. 465-466, July 24, 1981

16.   Armentano, "Pot Doesn't Rot Your Brain." *High Times*, No. 290, October, 1999

17.   Lyketsos et al., "Cannabis use and cognitive decline in persons under 65 years of age." *American Journal of Epidemiology*, Vol. 149, pp. 794-800, May 1, 1999

NOTES

18. *World Health Organization Project on Health Implications of Cannabis Use*, 1997
19. "U.S. Study: Marijuana might protect brain." Reuters, July 6, 1998
20. Radford, "Cannabis is stroke hope." *The Guardian* (UK), July 4, 1998

CHROMOSOME INTERFERENCE

1. "The health and psychological consequences of cannabis use," Chapter 6, National Drug Strategy Monograph No. 25, Australia
2. Hollister, "Health aspects of marijuana." Pharmacological Review, Vol. 38, No. 1, 1986
3. Bloch, et al., quoted in Hollister, op cit
4. World Health Organization Project on Health Implications of Cannabis Use, 1997

CONTAMINANTS

1. Hollister, "Health aspects of marijuana." *Pharmacological Review*, Vol. 38, No. 1, 1986
2. U.S. Department of Justice, Drug Enforcement Administration, *Cannabis Eradication in the Contiguous United States and Hawaii*
3. Edmunson, Project Leader, Environmental Analysis and Documentation, USDA/APHIS/PPD
4. Robberson, "U.S. pushes plan to apply poison on Colombian fields." *Dallas Morning News*, April 25, 1998
5. "Environmental Catch 22." Editorial, *The Toledo Blade*, July 31, 1999
6. McPartland, "Microbiological contaminants of marijuana." *Vermont Alternative Medicine*, 1994
7. Summary of the Testimony of Lester Grinspoon, MD before the Crime Subcommittee of the Judiciary Committee, U.S. House of Representatives, October 1, 1997
8. Grinspoon and Bakalar, *Marijuana: the Forbidden Medicine*. New Haven: Yale University Press, 1993
9. Young, DEA administrative law judge, Findings. *Marijuana Medicine and the Law*. Washington, DC: Galen Press, 1988

DEPENDENCE

1. Institute of Medicine, *Marijuana and Medicine: Assessing the Science Base.* Executive Summary, Washington DC: National Academy Press, 1999
2. Institute of Medicine, *op. cit.*
3. *World Health Organization Project on Health Implications of Cannabis Use*, 1997
4. Zimmer and Morgan, *Marijuana Myths: Marijuana Facts*. New York: The Lindesmith Center, 1997

DEPRESSION

1. "Big increase in rate of prescription drugs." Associated Press, February 18, 1998
2. "America's love affair with antidepressant drugs." *The Boston Globe*, October 17, 1999
3. Mikuriya, *Marijuana Medical Handbook*. Source: Schaffer Library of Drug Policy, www.druglibrary.org
4. Geiringer, "An overview of the human research studies on medical use of marijuana." 1994, Source: CANORML, www.norml.org/canorml/

5. Mikuriya, *op. cit.*

6. Hollister, "Health aspects of marijuana." *Pharmacological Review,* Vol. 38, No. 1, 1986

DIABETES

1. Maugh, "Inhaled form of insulin passes first test." *Los Angeles Times/Seattle Times,* June 17, 1998

2. Hollister, "Health aspects of marijuana." *Pharmacological Review,* Vol. 38, No. 1, 1986

3. Grinspoon, "Anecdotal surveys on diabetes." The Forbidden Medicine Website, www.rxmarihuana.com

4. Diabetic reports from Seattle and from the Sonoma Alliance for Medical Marijuana, 1998

5. "Pot garden's size brought case to court." Sonora Union Democrat (California), March 19, 1998

DIGESTIVE DISORDERS

1. Baron and Folan, "Ulcerative colitis and marijuana." *Annals of Internal Medicine,* Vol. 112, No. 6, p. 471, 1990

2. Grinspoon and Christine, "Marijuana and irritable bowel syndrome." The Forbidden Medicine Website, www.rxmarihuana.com

3. Grinspoon and Kluge, "Marijuana and Crohn's Disease." The Forbidden Medicine Website, www.rxmarihuana.com

DRY MOUTH

1. Mattes, Shaw, and Engelman, "Effects of cannabinoids (marijuana) on taste intensity and hedonic ratings and salivary flow of adults." *Chemical Senses,* Vol. 19, No. 2, pp. 125-140, 1994

EPILEPSY

1. Cuhna et al., "Chronic administration of cannabidiol to healthy volunteers and epileptic patients." *Pharmacology,* Vol. 21, 1980

2. Summary of the Testimony of Lester Grinspoon, MD before the Crime Subcommittee of the Judiciary Committee, U.S. House of Representatives, October 1, 1997

3. Martinez, "The Green Cross Lifevine." Green Cross Home Page, www.hemp.net/greencross/lifevine.html

4. Gieringer, "An overview of the human research studies on medical use of marijuana." 1994, Source: CANORML, www.norml.org/canorml/

5. Borger, "Marijuana substitute combats nerve gas." Scripps Howard News Service, Source: www.marijuananews.com, July 22, 1998

FERTILITY

1. Cone, Johnson, Moore, and Roache, "Acute effects of smoking marijuana on hormones, subjective effects and performance in male human subjects." *Pharmacology and Biochemical Behavior,* Vol. 24, No. 6, pp. 1749-1754, June, 1986

2. "The health and psychological consequences of cannabis use." Chapter 6, *National Drug Strategy Monograph No. 25,* Australia

3. Zimmer and Morgan, *Marijuana Myths: Marijuana Facts*. New York: The Lindesmith Center, 1997

GLAUCOMA

1. Randall, ed. Affidavit before Administrative Law Judge Francis L. Young of the US Drug Enforcement Administration, *Marijuana Medicine and the Law*. Washington, DC: Galen Press, 1988
2. Alliance for Cannabis Therapeutics, P.O. Box 19161, Sarasota, FL 34276
3. Merritt, Perry, Russell, and Jones, "Topical delta-9-tetrahydrocannabinol and aqueous dynamics in glaucoma." Journal of Clinical Pharmacology, (8-9 Suppl) pp. 467S-471S, August 21, 1981
4. Finn, "Cannabinoid investigations entering the mainstream." *The Scientist*, Vol. 12, No. 3, pp. 1-8, February 2, 1998
5. Randall, ed. op. cit.
6. Summary of the Testimony of Lester Grinspoon, MD before the Crime Subcommittee of the Judiciary Committee, U.S. House of Representatives, October 1, 1997
7. Merritt, Perry, Russell, and Jones, *op. cit.*
8. Green and Roth, "Ocular effects of topical administration of delta-9-tetrahydrocannabinol in man." *Archives of Opthalmology*. Vol. 100, No. 2, pp. 265-267, February 1992
9. Jay and Green, "Multiple-drop study of topically applied 1% delta-9-tetrahydrocannabinol in human eyes." *Archives of Opthalmology*, Vol. 101, No. 4, pp. 591-593, April 1993

HEPATITIS

1. *Consensus Statement of the European Association for the Study of Liver Disease.* International Consensus Conference on Hepatitis C, Paris, February 1999
2. *10 o'clock News*, FOX TV Channel 2 in San Francisco, June 23, 1998
3. Smith, Paithirana, Davidson, et al., *The origin of hepatitis C Genotypes*. Department of Medical Microbiology, University of Edinburgh Medical School, UK, 1997
4. *High Times*, p. 34, May 1998
5. Anecdotal reports from the Sonoma Alliance for Medical Marijuana, 1998

HUNTINGTON'S CHOREA

1. Consroe, Stern, and Snyder, "Effects of Cannabidiol in Huntington's Disease." *Neurology*, Vol. 36, (Suppl 1) p. 342, April 1986
2. "Marijuana and the brain: Scientists discover the brain's own THC." *Science News*, Vol. 143, No. 6, p. 88, February 6, 1993

IMMUNE RESPONSES

1. Hollister, "Health aspects of marijuana." *Pharmacological Review*, Vol. 38, No. 1, 1986
2. Hollister, "Marijuana and immunity." *Journal of Psychoactive Drugs*, Vol. 24, pp. 159-63, 1992
3. *World Health Organization Project on Health, Implications of Cannabis Use*, 1997
4. "The health and psychological consequences of cannabis use." Chapter 6, *National Drug Strategy Monograph No. 25*, Australia

5. Hollister, *op. cit.*

6. Finn, "Cannabinoid investigations entering the mainstream." *The Scientist,* Vol. 12, No. 3, pp. 1-8, February 2, 1998

7. Loveless, Harris, and Munson, "Hyporesponsiveness to the immunosuppressant effects of delta-8 tetrahydrocannabinol." *Journal of Immunopharmacology,* Vol. 3, No. 3-4, pp. 371-383, 1981

8. Zimmer and Morgan, *Marijuana Myths: Marijuana Facts.* New York: The Lindesmith Center, 1997

9. World Health Organization, *op. cit.*

INCARCERATION

1. NORML: www.norml.org

2. "FBI reports marijuana arrests exceed those for violent crime." *NORML News,* October 21, 1999

3. "New research published by Federation of American Scientists finds marijuana offenders crowding nation's prison and jails." *Marijuana Policy Project,* June 16, 1999

4. Kasirer, "Federal foolishness and marijuana." *New England Journal of Medicine,* January 30, 1997

5. Armentano, "Barry Frank Submits New Med-MJ Proposal." *High Times,* No. 287, July 1999

6. The Lindesmith Center, 888 Seventh Avenue, NY, NY 10106, www.lindesmith.org

7. Drug Policy Foundation, 4455 Connecticut Avenue, NW, #B-500, Washington, DC 20008, www.dpf.org

8. Johnston, "It's not the cancer that's killing her." November coalition discussion list, Spring, 1998, Source: www.november.org

9. Wishnia, "The IOM Medical-Marijuana Report." *High Times,* July, 1999

10. Egelco, "Federal judge orders closure of six Northern California pot clubs." Associated Press, May 14, 1998

11. Guara, "Legal hassles extinguishing pot clubs." *San Francisco Chronicle,* May 23, 1998

12. Minton, "US agents raid Peron's pot farm." *San Francisco Chronicle,* May 15, 1998, Also: San Francisco Examiner, May 1998

13. "Judge says jailed medical marijuana advocate must receive medication." Associated Press, August 1, 1998

14. Krassner, "Medical–Pot Ban Threatens Peter McWilliams' Life." *High Times,* July 1999

15. Gerhard, "Sense and Sinsemilla." *POZ Magazine,* June 1999

16. *California NORML Reports,* Vol. 23, March, 1999, Source: www.norml.org/canorml/

17. "Noam Chomsky on Renee Boje." Hemp-talk, September 6, 1999, Source: www.hemp.net

18. "National drug war leaders disregard science in medicinal marijuana debate." Marijuana Policy Project Press Release, April 20, 1999

19. Campbell III, ed. *Psychiatry News,* (Newspaper of the American Psychiatric Association) April 16, 1999, Source: www.appi.org/pnews

20. Quinn, "Court boosts medical marijuana clubs." Reuters, September 13, 1999

21. "Judge told to rethink marijuana ban." Associated Press, September 14, 1999

NOTES

INSOMNIA

1. Hollister, "Health aspects of marijuana." Pharmacological Review, Vol. 38, No. 1, 1986
2. Institute of Medicine, *Marijuana and Medicine: Assessing the Science Base.* Washington, DC: National Academy Press, 1999

INTRACTABLE HICCUPS

1. Gilson and Busalacchi, "Marijuana for intractable hiccups." Aurora Medical Group, Milwaukee WI 53212
2. Grinspoon, "Marijuana for intractable hiccoughs." The Forbidden Medicine Website, www.rxmarihuana.com

MARINOL

1. Calhoun SR, Galloway GP, Smith DE: J Psychoactive Drugs 1998; 10(2): 187-196, Quotation from: www.roxane.com
2. Randall, *Cancer Treatment and Marijuana Therapy,* Washington, DC: Galen Press, 1990
3. Ibid.
4. Vinciguerra, Moore, and Brennen, "Inhalation of Marijuana as an anti-emetic for chemotherapy." *New York State Journal of Medicine*, Vol. 88, pp. 525-527, 1988
5. Capaldina, Tashkin, Vilensky, and Talarico, "Does marijuana have a place in medicine?" *Patient Care*, Vol. 32, No. 2, p. 41, Jan. 1998
6. Wishnia, "The IOM Medical-Marijuana Report." *High Times*, July 1999
7. "Medical use of whole cannabis." Statement of the Federation of American Scientists, 1996

MENIERE'S SYNDROME

1. Martinez, "Meniere's syndrome." The Forbidden Medicine Website, www.rxmari-huana.com/Menière.htm

MENTAL ILLNESS

1. Hollister, "Health aspects of marijuana." Pharmacological Review, Vol. 38, No. 1, 1986
2. Conversations with double board-certified psychiatrist Francis Podrebarac, MD, 1999
3. Grinspoon and Wilson, "Marijuana and Bipolar Disorder." The Forbidden Medicine Website, www.rxmarihuana.com
4. Mikuriya, Marijuana Medical Handbook, 1998, Source: Schaffer Library of Drug Policy, wwwdruglibrary.org

MIGRAINE

1. Hannington, "Migraine, a blood disorder." *The Lancet*, Vol. 1, No. 501, 1978
2. Kaiser Permanente Public Information Release, KRCB radio in San Francisco, July 7, 1998
3. Volve, Dvilansky, and Nathan, "Cannabinoids Block Release of Serotonin from Platelets Induced by Plasma from Migraine Patients." *International Journal of Clinical Pharmacology*, Vol. 4, pp. 243-46, 1985

NOTES

4. Grinspoon, "Marijuana and Migraine." The Forbidden Medicine Website, www.rxmarihuana.com
5. Mikuriya, "Chronic Migraine Headache: five cases successfully treated with Marinol and/or illicit cannabis." Berkeley, 1991, Source: Schaffer Library of Drug Policy, www.druglibrary.org
6. Mikuriya, *Marijuana Medical Papers, 1839-1972.* Oakland: Medi-Comp Press, 1973
7. Grinspoon, *op. cit.*
8. Hodges, "Migraine." The Forbidden Medicine Website, rxmarihuana.com

MORTALITY

1. "Long term marijuana users suffer few health problems, Australian study indicates." *NORML News,* 1998, Source: www.norml.org
2. *The Brown University Digest of Addiction Theory and Application.* Vol. 15, No. 11, p. 7, November 1997, Electronic Collection: A20104041
3. "Deaths from drug errors rise sharply for outpatients." *The Seattle Times,* February 28, 1998
4. Annas, "Reefer madness—The federal response to California's medical-marijuana law." *The New England Journal of Medicine,* Vol. 337, No. 6, August 7, 1997

MULTIPLE SCLEROSIS

1. Grinspoon, "Multiple sclerosis." The Forbidden Medicine Website, www.rxmarihuana.com
2. Ellenberger, "Treatment of human spasticity with delta-9-tetrahydrocannabinol." Journal of Clinical Pharmacology, August 21, 1981
3. Ungerleider, Andrysiak, Fairbanks, Ellison, and Myers, "Delta-9-THC in the treatment of spasticity associated with multiple sclerosis." Advisory on Alcohol and Substance Abuse, Vol. 7, No. 1, pp. 39-50, 1987
4. "Cannabis: Look, Listen, Learn." Independent (UK), cannabis@independentco.org, 1998
5. Warden, "UK will speed up work on cannabis." The British Medical Journal, May 5, 1998
6. "MS patients to receive whole smoked marijuana in English trials." NORML News, July 30, 1998
7. Pertwee, Letters, The Scotsman, February 19, 1998, Source: Cowen, www.marijuananews.com
8. Meinck, Schonle, and Conrad, "Effects of cannabinoids on spasticity and ataxia in multiple sclerosis." Journal of Neurology, Vol. 236, pp. 120-122, 1989

MUSCLE SPASMS

1. Taber's Cyclopedic Medical Dictionary. Philadelphia: F.A. Davis Company, 1987
2. Petro and Ellenberger, "Treatment of human spasticity with delta-9-tetrahydrocannabinol." Journal of Clinical Pharmacology Vol. 21, pp. 413S-416S, 1981
3. Egli, Elsohly, Henn, and Spiess, "The effect of orally and rectally administered delta-9 tetrahydrocannabinol on spasticity: A pilot study with two patients." International Journal of Clinical Pharmacology, Vol. 34, No. 10, pp. 446-452, 1988
4. Dittrich, and Hofmann, "Delta-9-tetrahydrocannabinol shows antispastic and analgesic effects in a single case double-blind trial." Maurer, Henn, European Archive of Psychiatry and Neurological Science, Vol. 240, No. 1, pp. 1-4, 1990

5. Petro and Ellenberger, "References on multiple sclerosis and marijuana." 1998, Source: Schaffer Library of Drug Policy, www.druglibrary.org
6. Gieringer, "An Overview of human studies on medical use of marijuana." 1994, Source: CANORML. www.norml.org/canorml/
7. Petro, "Marijuana as a therapeutic agent for muscle spasm or spasticity" (case reports). 1980
8. Barnell, "Marijuana and spastic paraplegia." Source: Grinspoon, www.rxmarihuana.com
9. Jordan, "The luckiest woman on Earth." Highwitness News, High Times, No. 266, October, 1997
10. Stein, "Bits and Pieces." Geriatric Psychiatry News, Issue 3, No. 7, June/July 1999
11. "American Medical Association House of Delegates Report." December 9, 1997

NEURALGIA

1. "Testimony of Joanna McKee." Director of the Green Cross Patient Coop, on numerous television and public appearances in Washington State, 1992-1998. See: www.hemp.net/greencross/lifevine.html
2. Martinez, "Chronic pain." The Forbidden Medicine Website, www.rxmarihuana.com/martinez.html
3. Hotz, "Study confirms pot chemicals can relieve serious pain." *Los Angeles Times*, October 27, 1997
4. Finn, "Cannabinoid investigations entering the mainstream." *The Scientist*, Vol. 12, No. 3, pp. 1-8, February 2, 1998
5. Maurer, Henn, Dittrich, and Hofmann, "Delta-9-tetrahydrocannabinol shows antispastic and analgesic effects in a single case double-blind trial." *European Archive of Psychiatry and Neurological Science*, Vol. 240, No. 1, pp. 1-4, 1990

NEURODERMITIS

1. Randall, ed. *Marijuana Medicine and the Law*, Washington DC: Galen Press, 1988

NUTRITION

1. "Deferne and Pate, "Hemp Seed Oil: A source of valuable essential fatty acids." *Journal of the International Hemp Association*, Vol. 3, No. 1, pp. 4-7, 1996
2. Osborn, "Hempseed: Nature's Perfect Food?" *High Times*, pp. 36-39, 50-51, 55 and 56, April, 1992
3. Conrad, *Hemp For Health*. Rochester, VT: Healing Arts Press, 1997
4. Wirtshafter, "Why Hemp Seeds?" *Hemp Today*, Rosenthal, ed. Quick American Archives, 1994
5. Erasemus, *Fats that Heal, Fats that Kill*. BC, Canada: Alive Books, 1993
6. Label warning on "Pringles" package, 1998

OBSTETRICS

1. Mikuriya, *Marijuana Medical Papers, 1839-1972*. Oakland: Medi-Comp Press, 1973
2. Zimmer and Morgan, *Marijuana Myths: Marijuana Facts*. New York: The Lindesmith Center, 1997
3. "The health and psychological consequences of cannabis use." Chapter 6, *National Drug Strategy Monograph No. 25*, Australia

NOTES

4. Hollister, "Health aspects of marijuana." *Pharmacological Review*, Vol. 38, No. 1, 1986

5. Klein, Stein, and Hutzler, "Cigarettes, alcohol and marijuana: Varying associations with birthweight." *International Association of Epidemiology*, Vol. 16, No. 1, 1987

6. Dreher, Nugent, and Hudgkins, "Parental marijuana exposure and neonatal outcomes in Jamaica: An ethnographic study." *Pediatrics*, Vol. 93, No. 2, pp. 254-260, February 1994

7. Komp, "Babies born to Marijuana Smoking Mothers in Jamaica are Found to be Developmentally Superior." Source: www.snowcrest.net/stlight

8. Ward, "Birth of an Olympian." 1998

9. Wirtshafter, "A Hempen Birthing." Source: www.snowcrest.net/stlight

10. Reports from the Oakland Cannabis Co-op Meeting, May 1998

11. Mount, ed. "Introduction to cannabis and childbirth." Source: www.snowcrest.net/stlight

PSYCHOACTIVITY

1. Grinspoon, *Marijuana Reconsidered.* 3rd ed. San Francisco: Quick American Archives, 1971

2. Rossi, Kuehnle, and Mendelson, "Marijuana and mood in human volunteers." *Pharmacological Biochemistry and Behavior*, Vol. 4, pp. 447-453, 1978, Source: National Library of Medicine, www.ncbi.nlm.nih.gov/PubMed/

3. NORML, www.norml.org

4. Zimmer and Morgan, *Marijuana Myths: Marijuana Facts.* New York: The Lindesmith Center, 1997

5. Mathew, Wilson, Coleman, Turkington, and DeGrado, "Marijuana intoxication and brain activation in marijuana smokers." *Life Science*, Vol. 60, No. 23, pp. 2075-2089, 1997

6. *Taber's Cyclopedic Medical Dictionary.* Philadelphia: F. A. Davis Company, 1987

PSYCHOMOTOR SKILLS

1. Nelson, "A Critical review of the research literature concerning some biological and psychological effects of cannabis." Advisory Committee on Illicit Drugs, Cannabis and the Law in Queensland: Criminal Justice Commission of Queensland, Australia, 1993

2. Terhune et al., "The incidence and role of drugs in fatally injured drivers." Accident Research Group, Buffalo, NY, Report #DOT-HS-808-065

3. Rosenthal, Geiringer, Mikuriya, MD, Marijuana Medical Handbook: A Guide to Therapeutic Use. San Francisco: Quick American Archives, 1997

4. Robbe, Marijuana use and driving. Institute for Human Psychopharmacology, University of Limburg, 1994

5. Klonoff, "Marijuana and driving in real life situations." Science, Vol. 186, pp. 312-24, 1974

6. World Health Organization Project on Health Implications of Cannabis Use, 1997

7. London Free Press (Canada) May 8, 1997

REPLACEMENT OF MEDICATIONS

1. "Drug reactions kill more than 100,000." Associated Press, May 14, 1998

2. "Deaths from drug errors rise sharply for outpatients." *The Seattle Times*, February 28, 1998

3. Conversations with Rob Killian, MD, 1998

4. McWilliams, Testimony before the California Senate Medical Marijuana Distribution Summit, May 26, 1998, Source: California Senate Rules Committee

5. *Physician's Desk Reference of Pharmaceutical Products*. Montvale, NJ: Economics Data Production Company, 1994

6. "Parkinson's drug may spur hallucinations." Reuter's Health Information, May 11, 1998

7. Grinspoon, Science, 1997

8. *Physician's Desk Reference of Pharmaceutical Products*, op. cit.

9. "Painkiller can harm liver, FDA warns." Associated Press, February 11, 1998

10. Willman, "Fast-track diabetes drug tied to 33 deaths." *Los Angeles Times*, December 6, 1998

11. 6 o'clock News, ABC affiliate KGO TV in San Francisco, June 3, 1998

12. "New Jersey man claims Viagra vision problem caused car crash." Associated Press, July 28, 1998

13. Grinspoon, Affidavit before Judge Riccardo Martinez, King County Superior Court, WA, September 26, 1997

14. Eaton, "What you don't know can kill you." 1998

15. Grinspoon and Bakalar, "Marijuana: An old medicine of the future." 1997, Source. www.rxmarihuana,com

16. "Ask Andrew Weil." Health questions answered online, http//cgi.pathfinder.com/drweil/

17. Grinspoon and Bakalar, op. cit.

18. Letters, *High Times*, No. 273, May 1998

RESPIRATORY DISEASES

1. Ungerleider and Andrysiak, "Bias and the Cannabis researcher." *Journal of Clinical Pharmacology* (8-9 Suppl) pp. 153S-158S, August 21, 1981

2. Nelson, "A critical review of the research literature concerning some biological and psychological effects of cannabis." Advisory Committee on Illicit Drugs, Cannabis and the Law in Queensland: Criminal Justice Commission of Queensland, Australia, 1993

3. Edwards, M.D., Testimony before the National Academy of Sciences in New Orleans, January 1998

4. Mikuriya, Testimony during a medical necessity trial in the State of Washington, December, 1996

5. Abrams, Lindesmith Center Lecture, San Francisco, May 17, 1999

6. Gagnon, "Marijuana Less Harmful to Lungs than Cigarettes." *Medical Post* (Quebec), September 6, 1994

7. Edwards, M.D., *op. cit.*

8. Tashkin et al., "Effects of habitual use of marijuana and/or cocaine on the lung." Research Findings on Smoking of Abused Substances, *NIDA Research Monograph 99*, 1990

9. Abrams, *op. cit.*

10. Gagnon, op. cit.

11. Ibid.

12. Partnership For a Drug Free America, public information television release, May, 1998

13. California Research Advisory Panel, 1990

14. James, "Medical marijuana: Unpublished federal study found THC treated rats lived longer, had fewer cancers." AIDS Treatment News, January 17, 1997

15. "Health care use by frequent marijuana smokers who do not smoke tobacco." Western Journal of Medicine, Vol. 158, No. 6, pp. 596-601, June, 1993

16. Tashkin, "Is frequent marijuana smoking hazardous to health?" Western Journal of Medicine, Vol. 158, No. 6, pp. 635-637, June, 1993

17. Institute of Medicine, Marijuana and Medicine: Assessing the Science Base. Washington, DC: National Academy Press, 1999

18. Wishnia, "The IOM Medical-Marijuana Report." High Times, July 1999

19. Wu, Wright, Sassoon, and Tashkin, "Effects of smoked marijuana of varying potency on ventilatory drive and metabolic rate." American Revue of Respiratory Disease, Vol. 146, No. 3, pp. 716-721, 1992

20. US National Academy of Science quoted in, "The health and psychological consequences of c annabis use." Chapter 6, National Drug Strategy Monograph No. 25, Australia

21. "Heavy long term marijuana use does not impair lung function, says new study." Los Angeles Times, 22.May 3, 1997

22. "Deglamorising cannabis." Editorial, The Lancet, Vol. 346, No. 8985, p. 1241, November 11, 1995

23. Schlosser, "The Politics of Pot: A Government in Denial." Rolling Stone, March 4, 1999

24. Radford (Science Editor), "UN Study Suppressed." The San Francisco Guardian, February 19, 1998

25. Medical Marijuana on Town Meeting, KOMO TV, Seattle, March 9, 1997

26. Abrams, Lindesmith Center Lecture, San Francisco, May 17, 1999

27. Conversations with Elvy Musikka, federally authorized medical marijuana patient, 1997-1999

28. Institute of Medicine, Marijuana and Medicine, Assessing the Science Base. Washington, DC: National Academy Press, 1999

29. Abrams, op. cit.

30. "Lab tests show cannabis clubs' medical marijuana superior to government's." Press Release, CANORML, May 21, 1999, Source: www.norml.org/canorml/

SEXUAL ACTIVITY

1. Conrad, "Hemp: The Natural Flower of Health" Source: Mount, ed. "Cannabis and Childbirth," www.snowcrest.net/stlight/

SMOKING METHODS

1. Gieringer, "Marijuana Water Pipe and Vaporizer Study." MAPS Bulletin, 1996, CANORML, www.norml.org/canorml/

2. Wishnia, "The IOM Medical-Marijuana Report." High Times, July, 1999

3. Gieringer, op. Cit.

4. Mason, Perez-Reyes, Mcbay, and Folz, "Cannabinoid concentrations in plasma after passive inhalation of marijuana smoke." Journal of Analytical Toxicology, Vol. 4, pp. 172-174, July 7, 1983

5. In another study, passive exposure to 16 cannabis cigarettes over a six day period was shown to equal one cannabis cigarette actively smoked, Source: Cone and Johnson, "Contact highs and urinary cannabinoid excretion after passive exposure to marijuana smoke." Clinical Pharmacological Therapy, Vol. 40, No. 3, pp. 247-256, September 1986

NOTES

6. "Ask Andrew Weil." Health questions answered online, http//cgi.pathfinder.com/drweil/

STRESS REDUCTION

1. Mikuriya, *Marijuana Medical Handbook*. Source: Schaffer Library of Drug Policy, www.druglibrary.org
2. Guimares, "Anxiolytic effect of cannabidiol derivatives in the elevated plus-maze." *General Pharmacology*, Vol. 25, pp. 161-164, 1994
3. Zuardi et al., "Action of cannabidiol on the anxiety and other effects produced by delta-9 THC in normal subjects." *Psychopharmacology*, Vol. 76, pp. 245-250
4. Zuardi, et al., "Effects of ipsapirone and cannabidiol on human experimental anxiety." *Journal of Psychopharmacology*, Vol. 7, pp. 82-88
5. Undocumented case of Vietnam Veteran Fenly Crawford
6. Institute of Medicine, *Marijuana and Medicine: Assessing the Science Base*. Washington, DC: National Academy Press, 1999

STROKE AND HEAD TRAUMA

1. "High expectations for stroke drug." *Israel Business Today*, Vol. 8, No. 387, pp. 19, July 24, 1998
2. "Marijuana derivative benefits head trauma victims, human trials show." *Norml News*, October 8, 1998
3. Tye, "Marijuana product may aid in traumas." *Boston Globe*, October 7, 1998
4. "U.S. Study: Marijuana might protect brain." Reuters, July 6, 1998
5. Radford, "Cannabis is stroke hope." *The Guardian* (UK), July 4, 1998
6. Petro and Ellenberger, "Treatment of human spasticity with delta-9-tetrahydrocannabinol." *Journal of Clinical Pharmacology*, Vol. 21, pp. 413S-416S, 1981

TOLERANCE

1. Jones, Benowitz, and Herning, "Clinical relevance of cannabis tolerance and dependence." *Journal of Clinical Pharmacology*, (8-9 Suppl) p. 143S-152S, August 21, 1981
2. Jones, Benowitz, and Herning, *op. cit.*
3. Gettman, "The tolerance factor," High Times, No. 239, July 1995/"Tolerance to cannabinoids." www.hightimes.com/ht/new/petition/jgpetition/c3e.html
4. "The health and psychological consequences of cannabis use." Chapter 6, *National Drug Strategy Monograph No. 25*, Australia
5. Institute of Medicine, *Marijuana and Medicine, Assessing the Science Base*, National Academy Press, 1999

TOXICITY

1. Annas, "Reefer Madness—The federal response to California's medical-marijuana law." *The New England Journal of Medicine*, Vol. 337, No. 6, August 7, 1997
2. "Deaths from drug errors rise sharply for outpatients." *The Seattle Times*, February 28, 1998
3. American Psychiatric Association, *Desk Reference to the Diagnostic Criteria from DSM-3-R*
4. National commission on marijuana and drug abuse, 1972

5. Buckley, "Is marijuana fear a myth?" *National Review*, August 24, 1997

6. Hollister, "Health aspects of marijuana." *Pharmacological Review*, Vol. 38, No. 1, 1986

TREATING ADDICTION

1. Grinspoon, "Marijuana and heroin addiction." The Forbidden Medicine Website, www.rxmarihuana.com

2. Stein, "Bits and Pieces." *Geriatric Psychiatry News*, Issue 3, No. 7, June/July 1999

UPPER RESPIRATORY INFECTION

1. *Taber's Cyclopedic Medical Dictionary*. Philadelphia: F. A. Davis Company, 1987

2. *Canadian Government Commission of Inquiry into the Non-medical Use of Drugs*. Ottawa: Information Canada, 1972

3. Lamont, "Study Shows Marijuana Users as Healthy as the General Population." *Sydney Morning Herald*, February 18, 1997

4. "The health and psychological consequences of cannabis use." Chapter 6, *National Drug Strategy Monograph No. 25*, Australia

VIOLENCE

1. Gieringer, "An Overview of the human research studies on medical use of marijuana." 1994, Source: CANORML, www.norml.org/canorml/

2. *World Health Organization Project on Health Implications of Cannabis Use: A Comparative Appraisal of the Health and Psychological Consequences of Alcohol, Cannabis, Nicotine, and Opiate Use, II*. "The Probable Health Effects of Cannabis Use," 1997

3. Johnston, "Elderly mixing up television, reality: Study: Violent images on the tube disorienting seniors." *London Observer*, Source: *San Francisco Examiner*, May 26, 1998

4. Conversations with double board-certified psychiatrist Francis Podrebarac, MD, 1998-1999

ZELOTYPIA

1. *Taber's Cyclopedic Medical Dictionary*. Philadelphia: F. A. Davis Company, 1987

2. Martinez, "Chronic pain." The Forbidden Medicine Website, www.rxmarihuana.com/Martinez.html

3. The testimony of hundreds of medical marijuana patients interviewed by the author

4. Testimony before the California Senate Medical Marijuana Distribution Summit, May 26, 1998, Source: California Senate Rules Committee

5. Margaret Mead (1901-78) Scientist, explorer, writer, and teacher, Margaret Mead, worked in the Department of Anthropology at the American Museum of Natural History from 1926 until her death.

BIBLIOGRAPHY

6 o'clock News. ABC affiliate KGOTV in San Francisco, June 3, 1998

10 o'clock News. FOX TV Channel 2 in San Francisco, June 23, 1998

ABC Evening News. July 11, 1998

Abel, *Marijuana, The First Twelve Thousand Years.* New York: Plenum Publishing Corporation, 1980

Abrahamov, Abrahamov, and Mechoulam, "An efficient new cannabinoid anti-emetic in pediatric oncology." The Brettler Center for Medical Research, Hebrew University, Jerusalem, Source: *Journal of the International Hemp Association*, Vol. 2, No. 2, pp. 76-79

Abrams, Lindesmith Center Lecture, San Francisco, May 17, 1999

ACT UP, www.actupgg.org

"AIDS cases up dramatically among Americans 50 and up." *Newsday*, January 23, 1998

"AIDS drugs fail many." *Seattle Times*, September 30, 1997

Aigner, "Delta-9 tetrahydrocannabinol impairs visual recognition memory but not discrimination learning in rhesus monkeys." *Psychopharmacology*, Vol. 95, No. 4, pp. 507-511, 1988

Alliance for Cannabis Therapeutics, *ACT News.* Spring 1995, ACT, P.O. Box 19161, Sarasota, FL 34276

American Civil Liberties Union statement on marijuana prohibition, May, 1998

"American Medical Association House of Delegates Report." December 9, 1997, Source: Marijuana Policy Project, www.mpp.org

American Psychiatric Association, Desk Reference to the Diagnostic Criteria from DSM-3-R

Anecdotal reports from the Sonoma Alliance for Medical Marijuana, 1998

Annas, "Reefer madness—The federal response to California's medical-marijuana law." *The New England Journal of Medicine*, Vol. 337, No. 6, August 7, 1997

Armentano, "Barry Frank submits new Med-MJ proposal." *High Times*, No. 287, July 1999

—, "Pot Doesn't Rot Your Brain." *High Times*, No. 290, October, 1999

"Ask Andrew Weil." Health questions answered online, www.pathfinder.com/drweil/

Avakian, Horvath, Michael, and Jacobs, "Effects of marijuana on cardio-respiratory responses to submaximal exercise." Clinical Pharmacolocical Therapeutics, Vol. 6, pp. 777-781, 1979, Source: National Library of Medicine, www.ncbi.nlm.nih.gov/PubMed/

Axelrod, "Enzymatic synthesis of anandamide, an endogenous ligand for the cannabinoid receptor, by brain membranes." Laboratory of Cell Biology, National Institute of Mental Health, Bethesda MD, Source: *Proctor of the National Academy of Science*, Vol. 14, pp. 698-701, July 5, 1991

BIBLIOGRAPHY

Barnell, "Marijuana and spastic paraplegia." Source: Grinspoon, www.rxmarihuana.com

Baron and Folan, "Ulcerative colitis and marijuana." Annals of Internal Medicine, Vol. 112, No. 6, p. 471, Dartmouth-Hitchcock Medical Center, Hanover NH, March 15, 1990

Baum, Smoke and Mirrors. New York: Little, Brown and Company, 1997

Beltramo and Piomelli, "Functional role of high-affinity anandamide transport, as revealed by selective inhibition," Science, Vol. 277, No. 5329, p1094(4), 1997

Bertrand, Affidavit before Ontario Court (Canada) in the case of Christopher Clay. Source: www.hempnation.com/challenge/bertrand.html

"Big increase in rate of prescription drugs." Associated Press, February 18, 1998

Borger, "Marijuana substitute combats nerve gas." Scripps Howard News, July 22, 1998, Source: Cowen, www.marijuananews.com

The Brown University Digest of Addiction Theory and Application. Vol. 15, No. 11, p. 7, November 1997, Electronic Collection: A20104041

Buckley, "Is marijuana fear a myth?" National Review, August 24, 1997

California NORML Reports, Vol. 21, No. 3, 1997, CANORML, 2215-R Market St. #278, San Francisco, CA 94114, www.norml.org/canorml/

— , Vol. 23, March, 1999

California Research Advisory Panel, 1990

Campbell, The Power of Myth. New York: Doubleday, 1988

Campbell III, ed. Psychiatry News, (Newspaper of the American Psychiatric Association) April 16, 1999, Source: www.appi.org/pnews

"Cannabidiol: Wonder drug of the 21st century?" Source: Schaffer Library of Drug Policy, www.druglibrary.org

"Cannabis: Look, Listen, Learn." Independent (UK), cannabis@independentco.org, 1998, Source: Media Awareness Project, www.mapinc.org

Capaldina, Tashkin, Vilensky and Talarico, "Does marijuana have a place in medicine?" Patient Care, Vol. 32, No. 2, p. 41, January 1998

Castaneda et al., "THC does not affect striatal dopamine release: microdialysis in freely moving rats." 1991, Source: Gettman, Marijuana, Science, and Public Policy, 1991, www.norml.org/facts/mspp.shtml

"Chocolate and Cannabinol." The Washington Post, August 26, 1996

"CDC says a third of HIV cases untreated." Associated Press, September 26, 1997

"CMA backs removal of marijuana from Schedule I prohibitive status." NORML News, May 28, 1998, Source: www.norml.org (NORML, 1001 Connecticut Ave NW #1010, Washington, DC 20036) www.norml.org

Commission of Inquiry into the Non-medical Use of Drugs. Ottawa: Information Canada, 1972

Cone and Johnson, "Contact highs and urinary cannabinoid excretion after passive exposure to marijuana smoke." Clinical Pharmacological Therapy, Vol. 40, No. 3, pp. 247-256, September 1986

Cone, Johnson, Moore, and Roache, "Acute effects of smoking marijuana on hormones, subjective effects and performance in male human subjects." Pharmacology and Biochemical Behavior, Vol. 24, No. 6, pp. 1749-1754, June 1986

Conrad, "Hemp: The Natural Flower of Health." Source: Mount, ed. Cannabis and Childbirth, Source: www.snowcrest.net/stlight/

—, Hemp For Health. Rochester, Vermont: Healing Arts Press, 1997

—, Hemp, Lifeline to the Future. Los Angeles: Creative Xpressions Publications, 1993

BIBLIOGRAPHY

Consensus statement of the European Association for the Study of Liver Disease. International Consensus Conference on Hepatitis C, Paris, February 1999

Consroe, Stern, and Snyder, "Effects of Cannabidiol in Huntington's Disease." *Neurology* Vol. 36, (Suppl 1) p. 342, April 1986

Conversations with Rob Killian, MD, 1998

Conversations with Elvy Musikka, federally authorized medical marijuana patient, 1997-1999

Conversations with double board-certified psychiatrist Francis Podrebarac, MD, 1998-1999

Cowen, "Science journal reports that cannabinoid receptors located outside the brain and spine are affected when the skin or flesh is cut or hurt." July 16, 1998, Source: www.marijuananews.com

Cuhna, et al., "Chronic administration of cannabidiol to healthy volunteers and epileptic patients." *Pharmacology*, Vol. 21, 1980

"DEA Refers Marijuana Rescheduling Petition to HHS." The Law Offices of Michael Kennedy, NY, 1998

"Deaths from drug errors rise sharply for outpatients." *The Seattle Times*, February 28, 1998

"Deferne and Pate, "Hemp Seed Oil: A source of valuable essential fatty acids." *Journal of the International Hemp Association*, Vol. 3, No. 1, pp. 4-7, 1996

"Deglamorising cannabis." Editorial, *The Lancet*, Vol. 346, No. 8985, p. 1241, November 11, 1995

Devane, et al., *Science*, Vol. 258, pp. 1946-1949, 1992

Diabetic reports from Seattle and from the Sonoma Alliance for Medical Marijuana, 1998

"Diagnosis: smoke pot to relieve pain." *The University of Washington Daily*, May 1997

Dittrich, and Hofmann, "Delta-9-tetrahydrocannabinol shows antispastic and analgesic effects in a single case double-blind trial." Maurer, Henn, *European Archive of Psychiatry and Neurological Science*, Vol. 240, No. 1, pp. 1-4, 1990

Doblin and Kleiman, "Marijuana as anti-emetic medicine: A survey of oncologists experiences and attitudes." *Journal of Clinical Oncology* Vol. 9, pp. 1314-1319, 1991

"Doctors urges war on pain, more use of opium-based drugs." *Miami Herald*, January 29, 1998

Dreher, Nugent, and Hudgkins, "Parental marijuana exposure and neonatal outcomes in Jamaica: An ethnographic study." *Pediatrics*, Vol. 93, No. 2, pp. 254-260, February 1994, Schools of Nursing, Education, and Public Health, the University of Massachusetts, Amherst

Drug Enforcement Administration, Statement of Policy for the Use and Handling of Controlled Substances in the Treatment of Pain. 1998

Drug Policy Foundation, 4455 Connecticut Avenue, NW, #B-500, Washington, DC 20008, www.dpf.org

"Drug reactions kill more than 100,000." Associated Press, May 14, 1998

Eaton, "What you don't know can kill you." 1998, Source: Cowen, www.marijuananews.com

Edmunson, Project Leader, "Environmental analysis and documentation." USDA/APHIS/PPD, 4700 River Road, Unit 149, Riverdale, MD 20737-1238, Source: Colorado Hemp Initiative Project, P.O. Box 729, Nederland, CO, www.welcomehome.org/cohip.

Edwards, M.D., Testimony before the National Academy of Sciences in New Orleans, January 1998

BIBLIOGRAPHY

Egelco, "Federal judge orders closure of six Northern California pot clubs." Associated Press, May 14, 1998

Egli, Elsohly, Henn, and Spiess, "The effect of orally and rectally administered delta-9 tetrahydrocannabinol on spasticity: A pilot study with two patients." *International Journal of Clinical Pharmacology*, Vol. 34, No. 10, pp. 446-452, 1988

Ekert, Waters, Jurk, Mobilia, and Loughnan, "Amelioration of cancer chemotherapy-induced nausea and vomiting by delta-9-tetrahydrocannabinol." *Medical Journal of Australia*, Vol. 2 No. 12, pp. 657-659, December 15, 1979, Source: National Library of Medicine, www.ncbi.nlm.nih.gov/PubMed/

Ellenberger, "Treatment of human spasticity with delta-9-tetrahydrocannabinol." *Journal of Clinical Pharmacology*, August 21, 1981

"Environmental Catch 22." Editorial, *The Toledo Blade*, July 31, 1999

Erasemus, *Fats that Heal, Fats that Kill*. BC, Canada: Alive Books, 1993

Fackelmann, "Marijuana and the brain: scientists discover the brain's own THC." *Science News*, Vol. 143, No. 6, p. 88, February 6, 1993

"FBI reports marijuana arrests exceed those for violent crime." *NORML News*, October 21, 1999

"Federal report reignites medical marijuana debate." CNN, March 17, 1999

"Feds OK Marijuana Research." *Los Angeles Times*, May 21, 1999

Finn, "Cannabinoid investigations entering the mainstream." *The Scientist*, Vol. 12, No. 3, pp. 1-8, February 2, 1998

Formukong, Evans, and Evans, "Analgesic and anti-inflammatory activity of constituents of Cannabis sativa L." *Inflammation*, Vol. 12, No. 4 p. 361-371, 1988

"Functional role of cannabinoid receptors." Symposium Syllabus Press Conference, August 26, 1998

"Functional role of high-affinity anandamide transport, as revealed by selective inhibition." *Science*, Vol. 277, No. 5329, p. 1094(4), August 22, 1997

Gagnon, "Marijuana less harmful to lungs than cigarettes." *Medical Post* (Quebec), September 6, 1994

Gerhard, "Sense and Sinsemilla." *POZ Magazine*, June 1999

Gettman, "The tolerance factor." *High Times*, No. 239, July, 1995

—, *Drug Abuse, Cannabis and the Brain*. New York: Trans High Corporation, 1997, Source: www.hightimes.com/ht/tow/med/brain.html

—, "Marijuana an d the human brain." High Times, March 1995, Source: www.hightimes.com, also: www.umsl.edu/~rkeel/180/brain1.html

—, Marijuana, Science, and Public Policy. July 11, 1997, Source: www.norml.org/facts/mspp.shtml

—, "The Tolerance Factor." *High Times*, No. 239, July 1995

—, "Tolerance to Cannabinoids." Source: www.hightimes.com/ht/new/petition/jgpetition/c3e.html

Gieringer, "An overview of the human research studies on medical use of marijuana." 1994, Source: CANORML, www.norml.org/canorml/

—, "Marijuana Water Pipe and Vaporizer Study." *MAPS Bulletin*, 1996, Source: CANORML, www.norml.org/canorml/

Gifford, Gardner, and Ashby, "The effects of intravenous administration of delta-9-tetrahydrocannabinol on the activity of A10 dopamine neurons recorded in vivo in anesthetized rats." *Neuropsychopharmacology*, Vol. 36, No. 2, pp. 96-99, 1997, Source: National Library of Medicine, www.ncbi.nlm.nih.gov/PubMed/

Gilson and Busalacchi, "Marijuana for intractable hiccups." Aurora Medical Group, Milwaukee WI 53212, Source: Lancet, v351 n9098, January 24, 1998

BIBLIOGRAPHY

Green and Roth, "Ocular effects of topical administration of delta-9-tetrahydro-cannabinol in man." *Archives of Opthalmology*, Vol. 100, No. 2, pp. 265-267, February, 1992

Grinspoon, Affidavit before Judge Riccardo Martinez, King County Superior Court (WA), September 26, 1997

—, "Anecdotal surveys on diabetes." The Forbidden Medicine Website, www.rxmarihuana.com

—, "Marijuana and asthma." The Forbidden Medicine Website, www.rxmarihuana.com

—, "Marijuana and heroin addiction." The Forbidden Medicine Website, www.rxmarihuana.com

—, "Marijuana and migraine." The Forbidden Medicine Website, www.rxmarihuana.com

—, "Marijuana for intractable hiccoughs." The Forbidden Medicine Website, www.rxmarihuana.com

—, *Marijuana Reconsidered*, 3rd ed. San Francisco: Quick American Archives, 1971

—, "Medical use of marijuana: assessment of the science base." Review for Institute of Medicine, 1999

—, "Multiple sclerosis." The Forbidden Medicine Website, www.rxmarihuana.com

—, Science, 1997, Source: rxmarihuana.com

—, Summary of the Testimony of Lester Grinspoon before the Crime Subcommittee of the Judiciary Committee, U.S. House of Representatives, October 1, 1997

Grinspoon and Bakalar, "Marijuana: An old medicine of the future, 1997." Source: The Forbidden Medicine Website, www.rxmarihuana.com

—, *Marijuana, The Forbidden Medicine*. New Haven, Yale University Press, 1993

—, *Medical Uses of Illicit Drugs*. 1997, Source: Schaffer Library of Drug Policy, www.druglibrary.org

Grinspoon, Bakalar, Zimmer, and Morgan, "Marijuana Addiction." *Science*, Vol. 277, pp. 749, August 8, 1997

Grinspoon and Christine, "Marijuana and irritable bowel syndrome." The Forbidden Medicine Website, www.rxmarihuana.com

Grinspoon and Kluge, "Marijuana and Crohn's disease." The Forbidden Medicine Website, www.rxmarihuana.com

Grinspoon and Wilson, "Marijuana and bipolar disorder." The Forbidden Medicine Website, www.rxmarihuana.com

Guara, "Legal hassles extinguishing pot clubs." *San Francisco Chronicle*, May 23, 1998

Guimares, "Anxiolytic effect of cannabidiol derivatives in the elevated plus-maze." *General Pharmacology*, Vol. 25, pp. 161-164, 1994

Hannington, "Migraine, a blood disorder." *The Lancet*, Vol. 1, No. 501, 1978

"Hashish evidence is 1,600 years old." Associated Press, June 2, 1992

"The health and psychological consequences of cannabis use." Chapter 6, *National Drug Strategy Monograph No. 25*, Australia, Source: Schaffer Library of Drug Policy, www.druglibrary.org

"Health care use by frequent marijuana smokers who do not smoke tobacco." *Western Journal of Medicine*, Vol. 158, No. 6, pp. 596-601, June, 1993, Source: Geiringer, *Marijuana Health Mythology*, 1994, CANORML, www.norml.org/canorml/

"Heavy long term marijuana use does not impair lung function, says new study." *Los Angeles Times*, May 3, 1997

"High expectations for stroke drug." *Israel Business Today*, Vol. 8, No. 387, pp. 19, July 24, 1998

BIBLIOGRAPHY

High Times, p. 34, May 1998

"History of marijuana use: medical and intoxicant." from: *Marijuana, A Signal of Misunderstanding*, Report of the U.S. National Commission on Marijuana and Drug Abuse, 1972, Source: Schaffer Library of Drug Policy, www.druglibrary.org,

Hodges, "Migraine." The Forbidden Medicine Website, www.rxmarihuana.com

Holdcroft, et al., "Pain relief with oral cannabinoids in familial Mediterranean fever." *Anaesthesia*, Vol. 52, No. 5, pp. 483-486, May 1997

Hollister, "Health aspects of marijuana." *Pharmacological Review*, Vol. 38, No. 1, 1986

—, "Marijuana and immunity." *Journal of Psychoactive Drugs*, Vol. 24, pp. 159-63, 1992

Hooker and Jones, "Increased susceptibility to memory intrusions and the Stroop interference effect during acute marijuana intoxication." *Psychopharmacology*, Vol. 91, No. 1, pp. 20-24, 1987

Hotz, "Study confirms pot chemicals can relieve serious pain." *Los Angeles Times*, October 27, 1997

Institute of Medicine, *Marijuana and Medicine: Assessing the Science Base*. Washington, DC: National Academy Press, 1999

Jacobson, "US deaths from AIDS dropped 12% in period, study finds." *Dallas Morning Star*, February 28, 1998

James, "Medical marijuana: Unpublished federal study found THC treated rats lived longer, had fewer cancers." *AIDS Treatment News*, January 17, 1997

Jay and Green, "Multiple-drop study of topically applied 1% delta-9-tetrahydrocannabinol in human eyes." *Archives of Opthalmology*, Vol. 101, No. 4, pp. 591-593, April, 1993

Johnston, "Elderly mixing up television, reality: Study: Violent images on the tube disorienting seniors." London Observer, Source: *San Francisco Examiner*, May 26, 1998

Johnston, T., "It's not the cancer that's killing her." November Coalition discussion list, Spring, 1998, November Coalition: www.november.org

Jones, Benowitz, and Herning, "Clinical relevance of cannabis tolerance and dependence." *Journal of Clinical Pharmacology* (8-9 Suppl) p. 143S-152S, August 21, 1981, Source: National Library of Medicine, www.ncbi.nlm.nih.gov/PubMed/

Jordan, "The Luckiest Woman on Earth." Highwitness News, *High Times*, No. 266, October, 1997

"Judge says jailed medical marijuana advocate must receive medication." Associated Press, August 1, 1998

"Judge told to rethink marijuana ban." Associated Press, September 14, 1999

Kaiser Permanente Public Information Release. KRCB in San Francisco, July 7, 1998

Kasirer, ed. "Federal foolishness and marijuana." *New England Journal of Medicine*, January 30, 1997

Kaslow et al., from: *World Health Organization Project on Health Implications of Cannabis Use: A Comparative Appraisal of the Health and Psychological Consequences of Alcohol, Cannabis, Nicotine, and Opiate Use, II*. "The probable health effects of cannabis use." December 1997, Source: Schaffer Library of Drug Policy, www.druglibrary.org

Kleiman, *Against Excess: Drug Policy for Results*. New York: Basic Books, 1997

Klein, Stein, and Hutzler, "Cigarettes, alcohol and marijuana: varying associations with birthweight." *International Association of Epidemiology*, Vol. 16, No. 1, 1987

Klonoff, "Marijuana and driving in real life situations." *Science*, Vol. 186, pp. 312-24, 1974, Source: Gieringer, Marijuana Health Mythology, 1994, CANORML, www.norml.org/canorml/

BIBLIOGRAPHY

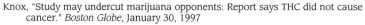

Knox, "Study may undercut marijuana opponents: Report says THC did not cause cancer." *Boston Globe*, January 30, 1997

Kolansky and Moore, 1971, Millman and Sbriglio, 1986, from: *World Health Organization Project on Health Implications of Cannabis Use: A Comparative Appraisal of the Health and Psychological Consequences of Alcohol, Cannabis, Nicotine, and Opiate Use, II*. "The probable health effects of cannabis use." December 1997, Source: Schaffer Library of Drug Policy, www.druglibrary.org

Komp, "Babies born to marijuana smoking mothers in Jamaica are found to be developmentally superior." Source: Mount, ed. www.Snowcrest.net/stlight/

Krassner, "Medical–pot ban threatens Peter McWilliams' life." *High Times*, July, 1999

"Lab Tests Show Cannabis clubs' medical marijuana superior to government's." Press Release, CANORML, May 21, 1999, www.norml.org/canorml/

Label warning on "Pringles" package, 1998

Laino, "Waiting to inhale: hemp for health?" MSNBC News, Spring 1998

Lamont, "Study shows marijuana users as healthy as the general population." *Sydney Morning Herald*, February 18, 1997

Latimer, "Highwitness News." *High Times*, No. 270, p. 30, February, 1998

Letter from American Cancer Society to CA Senator Vasconcellos, July 25, 1997

Letters, *High Times*, No. 273, May, 1998

Liegh, "Study brings breath of fresh air to pot smokers." Medical Tribune News Service, 1999

Lindesmith Center, 888 Seventh Avenue, NY, NY 10106, www.lindesmith.org

London Free Press (Canada), May 8, 1997

"Long term marijuana users suffer few health problems, Australian study indicates." *NORML News,* 1998, Source: www.norml.org

Loveless, Harris, and Munson, "Hyporesponsiveness to the immunosuppressant effects of delta-8 tetrahydrocannabinol." *Journal of Immunopharmacology*, Vol. 3, No. 3-4, pp. 371-383, 1981

Lyketsos, et al., "Cannabis use and cognitive decline in persons under 65 years of age." *American Journal of Epidemiology*, Vol. 149, pp. 784-800, May 1, 1999

"Marijuana and the brain: scientists discover the brain's own THC." *Science News*, Vol. 143, No. 6, p. 88, February 6, 1993

"Marijuana derivative benefits head trauma victims, human trails show." *NORML News*, October 8, 1998

Marijuana Policy Project, www.mpp.org

Marinol product information from Roxane Laboratories, Inc., Columbus, OH 43216, Source: Schaffer Library of Drug Policy, www.druglibrary.org

Martinez, "Chronic pain." The Forbidden Medicine Website, www.rxmarihuana.com/Martinez.html

—, "Meniere's syndrome," The Forbidden Medicine Website, www.rxmarihuana.com/Menière.htm

—, "The case of Joanna McKee." *The Green Cross Lifevine*: www.hemp.net/green-cross/lifevine.html

Mason, Perez-Reyes, Mcbay, and Folz, "Cannabinoid concentrations in plasma after passive inhalation of marijuana smoke." *Journal of Analytical Toxicology*, Vol. 4, pp. 172-174, July 7, 1983

Mathew, Wilson, Coleman, Turkington, and DeGrado, "Marijuana intoxication and brain activation in marijuana smokers." *Life Science*, Vol. 60, No. 23, pp. 2075-2089, 1997

BIBLIOGRAPHY

Mathre, ed. *Cannabis in Medical Practice*. North Carolina and London: McFarland and Company, 1997

Mattes, Shaw, and Engelman, "Effects of cannabinoids (marijuana) on taste intensity and hedonic ratings and salivary flow of adults." *Chemical Senses*, Vol. 19, No. 2, pp. 125-140, 1994

Maugh, "Inhaled form of insulin passes first test." *Los Angeles Times, Seattle Times*, June 17, 1998

—, "Similar effects found for pot, harder drugs." *Los Angeles Times*: Science Focus, June 27, 1997

Maurer, Henn, Dittrich, and Hofmann, "Delta-9-tetrahydrocannabinol shows antispastic and analgesic effects in a single case double-blind trial." *European Archive of Psychiatry and Neurological Science*, Vol. 240, No. 1, pp. 1-4, 1990

McKee, Director of the Green Cross Patient Coop, Testimony in news print and in numerous television and public appearances in Washington State, 1992-1998.

McPartland, "Microbiological contaminants of marijuana." *Vermont Alternative Medicine*, 1994, Source: *Journal of the International Hemp Association*, Vol. 1, pp. 41-44

McWilliams, "In the war on drugs, a Red Cross is just another target." www.petertrial.com

—, "Medical Marijuana and Me." Source: The Forbidden Medicine Website, www.rxmarihuana.com

—, Testimony before the California Senate Medical Marijuana Distribution Summit, May 26, 1998, Source: California Senate Rules Committee

"Medical marijuana: Doing the science." *Synapse*, 1998, Source: www.itsa.ucsf.edu/synapse/

"Medical marijuana." *Town Meeting*, KOMO TV, Seattle, March 9, 1997

"Medical use of whole cannabis." Statement of the Federation of American Scientists, 1996

"Medicinal Marijuana Briefing Paper 1997-98." *Marijuana Policy Project*, 1998, www.mpp.org

Meinck, Schonle, and Conrad, "Effects of cannabinoids on spasticity and ataxia in multiple sclerosis." *Journal of Neurology*, Vol. 236, pp. 120-122, 1989

"Mental fuzziness linked to marijuana." *Chicago Tribune*, February 21, 1996

Merritt, Perry, Russell, and Jones, "Topical delta-9-tetrahydrocannabinol and aqueous dynamics in glaucoma." *Journal of Clinical Pharmacology*, (8-9 Suppl) pp. 467S-471S, August 21, 1981

Mikuriya, "Chronic Migraine Headache: Five cases successfully treated with Marinol and/or illicit cannabis." Berkeley, 1991, Source: Schaffer Library of Drug Policy, www.druglibrary.org

—, *Marijuana Medical Handbook*. Source: Schaffer Library of Drug Policy, www.druglibrary.org

—, *Marijuana Papers*. Oakland: Medi-comp Press, 1973

—, Testimony during a medical necessity trial in the State of Washington. December, 1996

Minton, "US agents raid Peron's pot farm." *San Francisco Chronicle*, May 15, 1998, also: *San Francisco Examiner*, May, 1998

Morin, "Research into cannabinoids provides evidence that the use of marijuana to treat pain and nausea should not be so easily dismissed." May 1998, Source: Morin@Brown.edu

Mount, ed. "Introduction to cannabis and childbirth." www.snowcrest.net/stlight

BIBLIOGRAPHY

MS patients to receive whole smoked marijuana in English trials." *NORML News,* July 30, 1998

National Academy of Science, "The health and psychological consequences of cannabis use." Chapter 6, *National Drug Strategy Monograph No. 25,* Australia, Source: Schaffer Library of Drug Policy, www.druglibrary.org

National Cancer Institute, *Marijuana Use in Supportive Care for Cancer Patients.* Cancer Information Service, September 1997, Source: http://cancernet.nci/ NCI Toll-free: 1-800-4-CANCER

National Commission on Marijuana and Drug Abuse, 1972

"National drug war leaders disregard science in medicinal marijuana debate." Marijuana Policy Project Press Release, April 20, 1999, Source: www.mpp.org

Nature, Volume 363, May 20, 1993

Nelson, "A critical review of the research literature concerning some biological and psychological effects of cannabis." Advisory Committee on Illicit Drugs, Cannabis and the Law in Queensland: Criminal Justice Commission of Queensland, Australia, 1993. Source: Schaffer Library of Drug Policy, www.druglibrary.org

"New Jersey man claims Viagra vision problem caused car crash." Associated Press, July 28, 1998

"New lifesaving drugs explored as possible culprit." Associated Press, May 14, 1998

"New research Published by Federation of American Scientists finds marijuana offenders crowding nation's prisons and jails." *Marijuana Policy Project,* June 16, 1999

"New Scientist Special Report on Marijuana." *New Scientist,* February 21, 1998

"NIH Panelists Agree: Marijuana Is Safe and Effective Medicine." *MPP News,* August 4, 1997, Marijuana Policy Project, www.mpp.org

"Noam Chomsky on Renee Boje." *Hemp-talk,* September 6, 1999, www.hemp.net

NORML News, www.norml.org

Noyes and Baram, "Cannabis analgesia." *Comprehensive Psychiatry,* Vol. 15, No. 6, 1974

Noyes, Brunk, Baram, and Canter, "Analgesic effect of delta-9-tetrahydrocannabinol." *Journal of Clinical Pharmacology,* Vol. 2, No. 3, pp. 139-143, February 15, 1975

"NY State Legislator and head of NY Hospital's Department of Public Health Supports Medical Marijuana." Source: Cowen, www.marijuananews.com, January, 1998

Oakland City Council Resolutions on Medical Marijuana, June 1998

"Official Report Backs Medical Use of Marijuana." Reuters, March 17, 1999

Orr, Mckernan, and Bloome, "Anti-emetic effect of tetrahydrocannabinol Compared with placebo and prochlorperazine in chemotherapy-associated nausea and emisis." *Archives of Internal Medicine,* Vol. 140, No. 11, pp. 1431-1433, November 1980, Source: National Library of Medicine, www.ncbi.nlm.nih.gov/PubMed/

Osborn, "Hempseed: Nature's perfect food?" *High Times,* pp. 36-39, 50-51, 55 and 56, April 1992

"Painkiller can harm liver, FDA warns." Associated Press, February 11, 1998

Palella, et al., "Declining morbidity and mortality among patients with advanced human immunodeficiency virus." *New England Journal of Medicine,* Vol. 338, No. 13, p. 853, March 26, 1998

Pan, "On the origin of papermaking in the light of research on recent archeological discoveries." *Newsletter of the Friends of the Dard Hunter Paper Museum,* June 1987

"Parkinson's drug may spur hallucinations." Reuters Health Information, May 11, 1998

BIBLIOGRAPHY

Partnership For a Drug Free America, public information television release, May 1998

Pertwee, Letters, *The Scotsman*, February 19, 1998, Source: Cowen, www.marijuananews.com

Petro, "Marijuana as a therapeutic agent for muscle spasm or spasticity" (case reports). 1980, Source: D. J. Petro, MD, 1158 Lydig Ave, Bronx, NY 10461

Petro and Ellenberger, "References on Multiple Sclerosis and Marijuana." 1998, Source: Schaffer Library of Drug Policy, www.druglibrary.org

—, *"Treatment of Human Spasticity with delta-9-tetrahydrocannabinol." Journal of Clinical Pharmacology* Vol. 21, pp. 413S-416S, 1981, Source: Schaffer Library of Drug Policy, www.druglibrary.org

Physician's Desk Reference of Pharmaceutical Products, Montvale, NJ, Economics Data Production Co., 1994

Piomelli, "Functional role of high-affinity anandamide transport, as revealed by selective inhibition." *Science*, Vol. 277, No. 5329, p. 1094(4), August 22, 1997

"Planet Science: Marijuana special report," *New Scientist*, February 21, 1998

Portyansky, *Plant of a thousand uses (marijuana)*. Medical Economics Publishing, 1998, E. Collection: A20409468

Poster, Penta, Bruno, and Macdonald, "Delta-9-tetrahydrocannabinol in clinical oncology." *Journal of the American Medical Association*, Vol. 245, No. 20, pp. 2047-2051, May 22, 1988

"Pot chemical can relieve serious pain." *Los Angeles Times*, August 27, 1998

"Pot garden's size brought case to court." *Sonora Union Democrat* (California), March 19, 1998

"Pre-clinical studies show CT-3 reduces chronic and acute inflammation and reduces destruction of joints." BW HealthWire, January 1998, Source: Cowen, www.marijuananews.com

"Prisons can't cure drug problem, doctors tell US." *Miami Herald*, Herald Washington Bureau, March 18, 1998

Quinn, "Court Boosts Medical Marijuana Clubs." Reuters, September 13, 1999

Radford (Science Editor), "UN Study Suppressed." *The San Francisco Guardian*, February 19, 1998

Radford, T., "Cannabis is stroke hope." *The Guardian* (UK), July 4, 1998

Randall, Affidavit before Administrative Law Judge Francis L. Young of the US Drug Enforcement Administration, *Marijuana Medicine and the Law*. Washington, DC: Galen Press, 1988

—, *Cancer Treatment and Marijuana Therapy*. Washington, DC, Galen Press, 1990

—, ed. *Marijuana Medicine and the Law*. Washington DC: Galen Press, 1988, Alliance for Cannabis Therapeutics, P.O. Box 19161, Sarasota, FL 34276

"Researchers say many cancer patients suffer needless pain." Associated Press, June 17, 1998

"Researchers watch dopamine changes in brain of video game players." Associated Press, May 21, 1998

Robbe, "Marijuana use and driving." Institute for Human Psychopharmacology, University of Limburg, 1994

Robberson, "U.S. pushes plan to apply poison on Colombian fields." *Dallas Morning News*, April 25, 1998

Robinson, *The Great Book of Hemp*. Vermont: Park Street Press, 1996

Robson, "Cannabis as medicine: time for the phoenix to rise?" *British Medical Journal*, Vol. 316, No. 7137, p. 1034(2), April 4, 1998

Rosenthal, Geiringer, Mikuriya, MD, *Marijuana Medical Handbook: A Guide to Therapeutic Use*. San Francisco: Quick American Archives, 1997

BIBLIOGRAPHY

Rossi, Kuehnle, and Mendelson, "Marijuana and mood in human volunteers." *Pharmacological Biochemistry and Behavior*, Vol. 4, pp. 447-453, 1978, Source: National Library of Medicine, www.ncbi.nlm.nih.gov/PubMed/

Sallen, Zinburg, and Frei, "Anti-emetic effects of Delta-9 THC in patients receiving cancer chemotherapy." *New England Journal of Medicine*, Vol. 296, No. 16, 1975

San Francisco Chronicle, San Francisco Examiner, Associated Press, May 1998

Schaeffer, Andrysiak, and Ungerleider, "Cognition and Long Term Use of Ganja." *Science*, Vol. 213, pp. 465-466, July 24, 1981

Schlosser, "The politics of pot: A government in denial." *Rolling Stone*, March 4, 1999

Seeley, *Town Meeting*. KOMO TV 4 in Seattle, March 9, 1997

Smith, Paithirana, Davidson, et al., *The Origin of Hepatitis C Genotypes*. Department of Medical Microbiology, University of Edinburgh Medical School, UK, 1997

Statement of Dr. Richard Cohen, Consulting Medical Oncologist, California-Pacific Medical Center, San Francisco. Source: Californians for Medical Rights

Stein, "Bits and Pieces." Geriatric Psychiatry News, Issue 3, No. 7, June/July 1999

Stolberg, "Study finds elderly receive little pain treatment in nursing homes." June 17, 1998

"Study reveals pot chemicals can relieve serious pain." *Los Angeles Times*, October 27, 1998

"Study shows first downturn in AIDS." Associated Press, September 19, 1997

Symposium Syllabus: *Functional role of cannabinoid receptors*. Press Conference, August 26, 1998, Source: Medical Marijuana Magazine, www.marijuanam-agazine.com

Taber's Cyclopedic Medical Dictionary. Philadelphia: F. A. Davis Company, 1987

Tashkin, "Is frequent marijuana smoking hazardous to health?" *Western Journal of Medicine*, Vol. 158, No. 6, pp. 635-637

Tashkin et al., "Effects of habitual use of marijuana and/or cocaine on the lung." Research findings on smoking of abused substances, *NIDA Research Monograph 99*, 1990

Tashkin, Shapiro, Lee, and Harper, "Effects of smoked marijuana in experimentally induced asthma." *American Review of Respiratory Disease*, Vol. 112, 1975

Terhune et al., "The incidence and role of drugs in fatally injured drivers." *Accident Research Group*, Buffalo, NY, Report #DOT-HS-808-065, Source: National Technical Information Service, Springfield, VA 22161

"The health and psychological consequences of cannabis use." Chapter 6, *National Drug Strategy Monograph No. 25*, Australia

"The July 1995 Gettman/High Times petition to repeal marijuana prohibition: An extensive review of relevant legal and scientific findings." Source: www.hight-imes.com/ht/new/petition/jgpetition/index.html

The testimony of hundreds of medical marijuana patients interviewed by the author.

"Therapeutic possibilities in cannabinoids." Editorial, The Lancet, pp. 667-669, March 22, 1975

Tye, "Marijuana product may aid in traumas." Boston Globe, October 7, 1998

U.S. Code Congressional and Administrative News, 1970

U.S. Congress OTA, 1993, Source: Gettman, *Marijuana, Science and Public Policy*, www.norml.org/facts/mspp.shtml

U.S. Department of Justice, Drug Enforcement Administration, *Cannabis Eradication in the Contiguous United States and Hawaii*

—, *Statement of Policy for the Use and Handling of Controlled Substances in the Treatment of Pain*, 1998

BIBLIOGRAPHY

"U.S. study: marijuana is addictive." Reuters, March 31, 1998

"U.S. study: marijuana might protect brain." Reuters, July 6, 1998

"UN says HIV more widespread than thought." Associated Press, November 26, 1997

Undocumented case of Vietnam Veteran Fenly Crawford

Ungerleider and Andrysiak, "Bias and the cannabis researcher." *Journal of Clinical Pharmacology* (8-9 Suppl) pp. 153S-158S, August 21, 1981

Ungerleider, Andrysiak, Fairbanks, Ellison, and Myers, "Delta-9-THC in the treatment of spasticity associated with multiple sclerosis." *Advisory on Alcohol and Substance Abuse*, Vol. 7, No. 1, pp. 39-50, 1987

Vinciguerra, Moore, and Brennen, "Inhalation of Marijuana as an anti-emetic for chemotherapy." *New York State Journal of Medicine*, Vol. 88, pp. 525-527, 1988

Volve, Dvilansky, and Nathan, "Cannabinoids block release of serotonin from platelets induced by plasma from migraine patients." *International Journal of Clinical Pharmacology*, Vol. 4, pp. 243-46, 1985

Ward, "Birth of an Olympian." 1998

Warden, "UK will speed up work on cannabis." *The British Medical Journal,* May 5, 1998

Widener, "Study: Marijuana, morphine work on same area of brain," *The Seattle Times*, September 25, 1998

Williams, Boulton, de Pemberton, and Whitehouse, "Antiemetics for patients treated with antitumor chemotherapy." *Cancer Clinical Trials*, Vol. 3, No. 4, pp. 363-367, 1980, Source: National Library of Medicine, www.ncbi.nlm.nih.gov/PubMed/ , www.ncbi.nlm.nih.gov/PubMed/

Willman, "Fast-track diabetes drug tied to 33 deaths. LA Times, December 6, 1998

Wirtschafter, "A hempen birthing." Source: Mount, ed. www.Snowcrest.net/stlight/

—, "Why Hemp Seeds?" *Hemp Today,* Rosenthal, ed. Quick Trading Company, P. O. Box 429477, San Francisco, CA 94142, 1994

Wishnia, "The IOM medical-marijuana report." *High Times*, July, 1999

World Health Organization Project on Health Implications of Cannabis Use: A Comparative Appraisal of the Health and Psychological Consequences of Alcohol, Cannabis, Nicotine, and Opiate Use, II. "The probable health effects of cannabis use," 1997, Source: Schaffer Library of Drug Policy, www.druglibrary.org

Wu, Wright, Sassoon, and Tashkin, "Effects of smoked marijuana of varying potency on ventilatory drive and metabolic rate." *American Revue of Respiratory Disease*, Vol. 146, No. 3, pp. 716-721, 1992, Source: National Library of Medicine, www.ncbi.nlm.nih.gov/PubMed/

Young, DEA administrative law judge, Findings, Source: Randall, ed. *Marijuana Medicine and the Law*. Washington, DC: Galen Press, 1988

Zimmer and Morgan, *Marijuana Myths: Marijuana Facts.* New York: The Lindesmith Center, 1997

Zuardi et al., "Action of cannabidiol on the anxiety and other effects produced by delta-9 THC in normal subjects." *Psychopharmacology*, Vol. 76, pp. 245-250, Source: National Library of Medicine, www.ncbi.nlm.nih.gov/PubMed/

—, "Effects of ipsapirone and cannabidiol on human experimental anxiety." *Journal of Psychopharmacology*, Vol. 7, pp. 82-88, Source: National Library of Medicine, www.ncbi.nlm.nih.gov/PubMed/

About the Author

Martin Martinez grew up in rural Upstate New York. Early memories include accompanying his grandmother, a Methodist minister, on her frequent visits to hospitalized parishioners. Years of horsemanship were followed by a strong focus on art and music. By the age of 18 Martin was running a home business producing custom knitwear-managing a small retail outlet and a handful of employees. Later, along with a demanding career in business and real estate management, he also managed large construction and painting projects. At the age of 26, Martin Martinez was riding a motorcycle when an oncoming automobile veered into his lane and the two vehicles collided. A combined speed of 60 miles per hour propelled him 40 feet from the point of impact. He was not expected to survive. But he lived, kept alive for 30 days in the intensive care unit, after which he was hospitalized for months. He was expected to remain attached to a primary care facility for the rest of his life.

Doctors treated his condition with up to 10 milligrams of morphine every 7 minutes, 24 hours per day. Martin was severely crippled not only by his extensive orthopedic and neurological injuries, but also by the powerful effects of opiate painkillers. However, during the following years he substituted cannabis, which he used on a daily basis, for the opiate narcotics and other drugs. Ten years later, after a regimen of physical therapy and medical marijuana, Martin had recovered sufficiently not only to return to art school, take on several literary projects, and go back to real estate management, but also to perform major carpentry work on a full-time basis—to the amazement of all witnesses.

Managing and developing several residential properties in Seattle, Washington, Martin was cautious to conceal his use of marijuana from clients and tenants. In 1996, however, he was arrested for "manufacturing" marijuana, the mild herbal medication that made possible his unlikely recovery from horrendous trauma. Martin's medical necessity trial of 1997 ended in a hung jury of eight to four in favor of acquittal, but was followed by a second arrest: again, for "manufacturing" medical marijuana in his home. Twenty-two months of legal battles culminated in several weeks of fierce protest by hundreds of concerned citizens in Washington and other states. Five separate physicians testified on the validity of Martin's medical use of marijuana. With strong public outcry, and an advancing shift in public opinion on medical marijuana, the State of Washington settled the case with some sense of compassion. Martin Martinez was not jailed for his horticultural crimes. In the following year, Washington became one of six American states to enact laws protecting medical marijuana patients from criminal prosecution.

Martin Martinez now divides his time between writing and ministering to other severely ill patients.

About Dr. Podrebarac

Francis Podrebarac, M.D., was born in Wichita, Kansas, to a mother and father who both practiced medicine in the old tradition of direct patient care. In a home governed by intelligent compassion, Francis learned basic principles of medical care long before graduating from the University of Kansas School of Medicine at Wichita, where he also did his residency. He did a fourth year residency, with a fellowship, in geriatric psychiatry and geriatric research at the University of Washington Department of Psychiatry and Behavioral Sciences in Seattle, Washington, after which he became staff psychiatrist and treatment team leader at Washington State Hospital in Tacoma, Washington. There he dedicated eighty percent of his professional time to direct patient care. Dr. Podrebarac has always placed care of the patient above all other considerations, even at the risk of professional peril. In fact, a State of Washington Supreme Court ruling bears his name for exposing patient neglect at a geriatric facility in Washington State.

A lifetime devoted to patient care was interrupted by life-threatening intestinal cancer and infection with the AIDS virus. Five years later, Dr. Podrebarac is certain that medical marijuana was the key factor that enabled him to survive advanced stages of cancer, and he continues to credit medical marijuana as crucial to the survival of many AIDS patients. Having outlived his physicians' expectations, Dr. Podrebarac is now semi-retired, though he remains devoted to direct patient care. Additionally, Dr. Podrebarac is a vocal activist who helped draft the new medical marijuana law in Washington State.

INDEX

A

abdominal pain, x, 2. *See also* constipation; digestive disorders; intestinal cramps

abuse. See addiction; drug abuse; gateway theory

Acquired Immune Deficiency Syndrome. *See* AIDS

ACT UP, 22

addiction, 29–32, 49, 57, 113, 119, 126, 130–131
    definition of, 29
    and narcotics, 33
    treating, 115

adverse effects. *See* side effects.

AIDS (Acquired Immune Deficiency Syndrome) ix, 14, 21–28, 70–71, 76, 129
    and anorexia, 15, 23
    and cancer, ix, 23
    and chemotherapy. *See* chemotherapy and AIDS
    effects of, 22
    and medical marijuana legalization, 17, 23, 28, 120
    and mortality, 22, 81–82

and race, 22
    risk groups, 21
    in US, 21
    See also HIV; wasting syndrome

AIDS cocktail, x, 22

allergies to cannabinoids, 71. *See also* immune responses

American Medical Association, 11, 12, 27, 33, 42–43, 84, 97

American Psychiatric Association, 58, 74

analgesia, 32–36, 85, 93. *See also* pain management

anectdotal evidence, xii, 23, 61, 68, 73, 79, 80, 85, 90, 111
    as scientific evidence, 17–18

anorexia, 37, 61
    in AIDS patients, 15, 23

antibiotic properties, 37–38

anticonvulsant effects, 10, 39–40

antiemetic properties. *See* nausea; Marinol as antiemetic

antimotivational syndrome, 38–39

drug comparisons with
marijuana:
alcohol, 60, 65, 94, 117, 131
codeine, 36, 84
multiple drugs, x, xii, 16, 30,
33, 49, 53, 58, 99–100,
117, 119, 126, 131
painkillers, 35, 36, 84, 85,
93
prescription drugs, 44, 59,
62–63, 75, 82–84, 97, 98,
127
tobacco, 65, 101–4, 130
Drug Enforcement
Administration (DEA), x, 32,
33, 55, 120, *See also* policy
drug testing, 92, 96, 108
drug war, 55, 73, 74, 121
policy, 13, 27, 110
rhetoric, ix, 14, 26–27
dry mouth, 61–62. *See also* side
effects
dystonia, 62. *See also*
Huntington's chorea;
muscle spasms

E

elderly persons and medical
marijuana use, 57, 128
epilepsy, 62–63. *See also* anticonvulsant effects

F

fertility, 63–64, 112
Food and Drug Administration
(FDA), 22, 25, 44, 86, 99

G

ganja, 7
gateway theory, ix, x, 65, 119,
131. *See also* addiction;
dependence and marijuana;
drug abuse; drug compar-
isons with marijuana
glaucoma, 66–67
government. *See also* Drug
Enforcement
Administration; legalization;
policy
federal, ix, 13,
as provider of medical marijuana, 16–17, 105, 106
restrictions on study, 17, 25,
27, 43, 45, 76, 105, 122

H

hallucinations, x, 91–92. *See
also* psychoactivity
hangover effect, 75, 92
hashish, 7, 101
headaches, 90
as adverse effect of
narcotics, 33
See also migraine
headaches
head trauma, 52, 83–84,
110–111
hemp, 1, 2, 9, 12, 89, 108
and marijuana, 1
fiber industry, 11, 12, 13, 89
hepatitis, 67–68
hiccups. *See* intractable
hiccups

worldwide trends. *See* statistics, worldwide trends

Z

zelotypia, 118
zero tolerance, 95, 110